Exploring English
through Health Care Issues
toward a Better Life

英文ニュースで学ぶ
健康と
ライフスタイル

YOSHIFUMI TANAKA
田中芳文
【編著】

講談社

英文ニュースで学ぶ　健康とライフスタイル

あらかじめご了承ください

・本書は全国の大学・専門学校で教材使用されているため、問題の解答や日本語訳は付属していません。

・先生用にCD（非売品）が用意されています。（収録箇所：各Unitの◎の部分）

・音声の一般提供は行っておりません。

はじめに

　日本が超高齢化社会を迎えた今，病気にならないように，いかにして健康的な生活を送るかということが，私たちの重要な関心事となっています。そして，日常生活においては，新聞・雑誌やテレビ・ラジオ，あるいはインターネットなどのメディアを通して，私たちが「健康」や「ライフスタイル」に広く関連のあるトピックを扱うニュースに触れる機会が飛躍的に増加しています。本書は，そのような内容の英文ニュースを読みながら英語を学習するためのテキストです。

　VOA（Voice of America）を中心に，そのほかThe Japan TimesやThe Guardianなどに掲載されたニュースを本文として使用しています。その英文には，なるべく辞書を引かなくても読み進めることができるように，できるだけ多くの脚注を付けました。練習問題は，A（本文の内容理解を確認するための問題），B（本文に出てくる重要表現が含まれた英文を聴いて書き取る問題），C（本文に出てくる重要表現や構文を使った並べかえ英作文問題），D（本文に出てくる「健康」や「ライフスタイル」関連の語彙の問題）から構成されています。

　本書を利用することによって，「健康」や「ライフスタイル」に関するさまざまなトピックに対するみなさんの知識が深まると同時に，英語の学力が向上することを願っています。

　最後に，本書出版の意義にご理解をいただいた講談社サイエンティフィクに敬意を表しますとともに，出版のためにご尽力くださった同社の小笠原弘高さんにこころより感謝申し上げます。

2016年盛夏

編著者

執筆者一覧

飯島睦美
群馬大学大学教育・学生支援機構大学教育センター　教授 (4)

片岡由美子
愛知県立大学看護学部　准教授 (3)

ケネス・スレイマン
天使大学看護栄養学部　准教授 (英文校正)

鈴木繁雄
桜美林大学　名誉教授 (9)

※田中芳文
島根県立大学人間文化学部　教授 (2, 13)

長坂香織
山梨県立大学看護学部　教授 (12)

名木田恵理子
川崎医療短期大学　教授 (1, 7)

廣渡太郎
日本赤十字秋田看護大学看護学部　教授 (5, 8)

マユーあき
島根県立大学人間文化学部　教授 (6)

目時光紀
天使大学看護栄養学部　准教授 (11)

山内　圭
新見公立大学健康科学部　教授 (14, 15)

山﨑麻由美
神戸常盤大学保健科学部　教授 (10)

五十音順、※は編著者。（　）内の数字は担当Unit。

目次 CONTENTS

はじめに ……………………………………………………………………………… iii

Unit 1 温暖化対策で世界を健康に ……………………………………………… 1
WHO: Climate Change Brings New Health Threats
Experts: Climate Change Is a Medical Emergency

Unit 2 肥満という流行病 …………………………………………………………… 7
Researcher: Obesity Poses Complex Problem

Unit 3 「尊厳死」か「自殺ほう助」か？
──米国の終末期医療の側面 ………………………………………… 13
In US, Growing Push for 'Aid in Dying' for Terminally Ill

Unit 4 医療現場におけるロボット活躍の可能性 …………………………… 19
Robot Helps Heal Human Muscle Damage
Robot Scientist Helps Design New Drugs
Damaged Robots Learn to Make Changes to Keep Working

Unit 5
産科フィスチュラ撲滅をめざして 26
UN Report Links Progress with Efforts to End Fistula

Unit 6
断食が心身にもたらす効用 32
Jeanette Winterson: Why I Fasted for 11 Days

Unit 7
偏った食習慣が病気を招く：味覚障害からうつ病まで 38
Low Zinc Levels Tied to Dulled Sense of Taste: Unbalanced Eating Habits May Cause Zinc Deficiency
Unbalanced Eating Habits, a Cause of Depression

Unit 8
エボラ出血熱生存者たちの苦しみ 45
Many Ebola Survivors Struggling with Ailments

Unit 9
誰でもできる健康レシピ 52
Herbs and Spices May Improve Your Health

Unit 10
成長を続けるティーンエイジャーの脳 58
Understanding the Teen Brain Key for Better Parenting

Unit 11
血圧と食生活の関係 64
Dietary Changes Help Lower Blood Pressure
Study: Packaged Food Contains Unhealthy Levels of Salt

Unit 12
伝統医療と現代医学の統合 71
Americans Turn to Complementary, Alternative Medicine for Pain Relief
WHO Pursuing Update on Global Strategy for Traditional Medicine

Unit 13
卵巣がんとの闘い 78
Battling Ovarian Cancer: Clara's Story

Unit 14
"最期のとき"をどう決めるか 85
A Woman Ends Her Pain, But the Law Just Won't Let Go
Exit International Member's Death Prompts Victoria Police to Suspect Assisted Suicide

Unit 15
「老年植民地主義」または「姥捨て貿易」か？ 93
Some with Alzheimer's Find Care in Far-Off Nations

Unit 1

温暖化対策で世界を健康に

WHO: Climate Change Brings New Health Threats

Voice of America, August 27, 2014

track 01

The World Health Organization (WHO) warned Wednesday that major killer diseases will spread and health problems will worsen with climate change.

The WHO, which is holding the first global conference on health and climate in Geneva, urged nations to act quickly to reduce the emissions of greenhouse gases, which lead to climate change.

Although some countries could see localized benefits from global warming -- cold countries could experience fewer winter deaths due to more temperate weather as well as increased food production -- the WHO says overall health effects are likely to be overwhelmingly negative.

Maria Neira, director of the Public Health, Environmental and Social Determinants of Health Department at WHO, says seven million people die prematurely every year because of air pollution, but that number can be cut.

"We can reduce dramatically non-communicable diseases, cardiovascular diseases, heart disease, respiratory diseases, by promoting, for instance a more sustainable, low-carbon society where instead of using very pollutant and solid fuels," Neira said, "we will move into a more sustainable energy consumption and, therefore, by doing so, we will obtain plenty of benefits for our health."

Notes:

the World Health Organization (WHO)／世界保健機関　climate change／気候変動　threat／脅威　warn／警告する　killer disease／致死の(命にかかわる)病気　worsen／悪化する　conference／会議　urge A to ~／Aに~するよう強く促す　emission／放出，排出　greenhouse gas／温室効果ガス　benefit／利益　global warming／地球温暖化　due to ~／~が原因で　temperate weather／温帯気候　A as well as B／Bだけでなく A も　overall／全体の，総合的な　be likely to ~／~しそうである　overwhelmingly／圧倒的に　negative／マイナスの　the Public Health, Environmental and Social Determinants of Health Department／公衆衛生環境局(公衆衛生，環境，健康の社会的決定要因担当局)　prematurely／早すぎて　because of ~／~が原因で　air pollution／大気汚染　non-communicable disease／非感染性疾患(がん，糖尿病，呼吸器・循環器系疾患など)　cardiovascular disease／循環器疾患　respiratory disease／呼吸器疾患　for instance／たとえば　sustainable／持続可能な　low-carbon／低炭素の　instead of ~／~のかわりに　pollutant／汚染物質　solid fuel／固形燃料　plenty of ~／たくさんの~

The health community is working to improve surveillance to control infectious diseases and she says deadly diseases such as cholera, malaria and dengue are highly sensitive to weather and climate.

Recent WHO figures show that climate change already causes tens of thousands of deaths every year from shifting patterns of disease and extreme weather events, such as heat waves and floods.

Climate change is expected to cause approximately 250,000 additional deaths every year between 2030 and 2050 due to heat exposure, diarrhea, malaria, and childhood under-nutrition.

Alistair Woodward, the coordinating lead author of the health chapter of the Fifth Assessment Report of the Intergovernmental Panel on Climate Change, says there is opportunity for positive change.

"Transport systems, which produce maybe a quarter of the greenhouse emissions, are unhealthy and damaging to the environment in many ways," Woodward said. "If we could increase the use of active transport, our estimates are putting people on bikes, the benefit cost ratio is maybe 10 to one … Air pollution … If we put in practice what we know about ways of reducing black carbon emissions, diesel filters, plain cook stoves, for example, then we could probably save around two million premature deaths a year."

The WHO notes that climate change also has serious economic consequences. The U.N. agency says the direct damage costs to health is estimated to be between $2 billion and $4 billion a year by 2030.

Notes:

surveillance／監視,調査　infectious disease／感染症　deadly disease／命にかかわる病　A such as B／BのようなA　cholera／コレラ　malaria／マラリア　dengue (fever)／デング熱　be sensitive to 〜／〜に敏感である　figures／統計,データ　tens of thousands of 〜／数万の〜　extreme weather event／異常気象事象　heat wave／熱波　flood／洪水　approximately／およそ　heat exposure／高温曝露（暑気あたり）　diarrhea／下痢　under-nutrition／低栄養　the Intergovernmental Panel on Climate Change／気候変動に関する政府間パネル（国際的な専門家でつくる，地球温暖化についての科学的な研究の収集・整理のための政府間機構。数年おきに地球温暖化に関する Assessment Report（評価報告書）を発行）　opportunity／好機,チャンス　transport system／輸送システム　a quarter／4分の1　active transport／能動輸送　estimate／見積もり　put A on B／A(人)をBにのせる　benefit cost ratio／費用対効果比　put in practice／実行する　black carbon／黒色炭素（温室効果ガスとして，CO_2，メタンガスの次に影響力がある）　diesel filter／ディーゼルフィルター（排ガスに含まれる微粒子を捕集するフィルター）　plain cook stove／簡易（調理用）コンロ　premature death／早死（若年死亡）　consequence／（必然的）結果　billion／10億

Experts: Climate Change Is a Medical Emergency

Voice of America, August 19, 2015

track 02

　　Health and medical experts gathered in Washington this week for talks on climate change and public health. They met at the White House. The meeting was held a day after the U.S. Environmental Protection Agency released a report on climate change. The report explores the health and economic reasons for lowering climate changing emissions. The findings are similar to those of an independent research group, the Lancet Commission on Health and Climate.

　　The Lancet Commission report says the effects of climate change could threaten the past 50 years of gains in public health. Commission project leader Nicolas Watts says the changes in Earth's climate have led to weather extremes. The extremes can create public health risks that he considers very dangerous and unacceptable.

　　Mr. Watts says the changes have led to less rainfall, and this has been linked to a drop in agricultural productivity. The reduced productivity has led, in turn, to an increase in malnutrition, especially among children.

　　Studies have linked climate change to an increased likelihood of flooding in some areas. Mr. Watts says floods are linked to a rise in the rates of infectious diseases, cholera and problems that result from a breakdown of waste treatment systems. He also notes that the world is getting hotter. In 2003, 70,000 people in Europe died because of higher than normal temperatures. "And those sorts of events are expected to increase in frequency and severity as time goes on." Nicholas Watts spoke to VOA on Skype.

　　The World Health Organization has warned that serious action is required to reduce global warming emissions. If the reduction does not happen, the WHO says, there will

Notes:

emergency／緊急事態　public health／公衆衛生，全住民の健康　be held／開催される　the U.S. Environmental Protection Agency／米国環境保護局　explore／探究する，調査する　emission／放出物質，排出物質　findings／調査結果　be similar to ～／～と似ている　Lancet Commission on Health and Climate (Change)／健康と気候変動に関するランセット委員会　threaten／脅かす　lead to ～／（結果として）～につながる，～を招く　weather extremes／異常気象　rainfall／降雨　be linked to ～／～と関係している　agricultural productivity／農業生産性　in turn／今度は，次には　malnutrition／栄養不良　likelihood／可能性，見込　flooding／洪水　infectious disease／感染症　cholera／コレラ　result from ～／～から起こる　breakdown／機能停止　waste treatment system／廃棄物処理システム　because of ～／～が原因で　temperature／温度　those sorts of ～／そういった類の～　frequency／頻度　severity／ひどさ　as time goes on／時が経つにつれ

be serious results. By 2030, almost 250,000 people will die every year from the effects of global warming.

But the Lancet Commission report also describes growing evidence of the effects of actions to slow climate change. It says that such actions are good for global health. Outdoor air pollution is linked to almost three million deaths worldwide. About 1.2 million of those deaths are in China alone. Mr. Watts says a move from coal-fueled power plants to renewable energy, such as sunlight and wind power, can greatly reduce that danger.

He also says that moving to renewable energy will lead to fewer people being treated in hospitals and a drop in health care costs. He says this will, in turn, help struggling health budgets. Suggesting that people use active forms of transportation like bicycles may help reduce diabetes and obesity, he adds.

The Lancet Commission suggests several ways to deal with climate change. They include closing coal power plants, increasing the use of renewable energy, investing in health systems and agreeing to support a global climate treaty. World leaders are expected to meet in Paris in December to sign that measure. Mr. Watts says that politics and complex issues will be debated. But no matter what, he says, the treaty is about public health.

"When you start to do that you realize that actually the responses to climate change aren't things that are necessarily hurt and they are not necessarily things that are going to result in a lower quality of life. In fact, most of what you want to do to respond to climate change is good for public health and it is actually a much brighter future."

Mr. Watts hopes the Commission's report helps unite health care experts behind a global treaty. He hopes that the treaty can respond to the risks of climate change. "What is good for the planet," he adds, "is good for patient care."

Notes:

die from ～／～が原因で死ぬ　describe／述べる，記述する　evidence／証拠　outdoor air pollution／屋外の大気汚染　coal-fueled power plant／石炭燃料による発電所　renewable energy／再生可能エネルギー　health care cost／医療費　struggling／苦労している　health budget／医療予算　active form of transportation／能動輸送　diabetes／糖尿病　obesity／肥満　deal with ～／～に対処する　coal power plant／石炭発電所　invest／投資する　treaty／条約，条約議定書　measure／法案　politics／政治　debate／議論する　no matter what／たとえ何があろうと　not necessarily ～／必ずしも～でない　quality of life／生活の質　in fact／実際には，もっとはっきりいえば　unite／団結させる

練習問題

A 本文の内容に合うように，各英文の（ ）内に入る最も適切な語句をそれぞれ1つずつ選びなさい。

1. Non-communicable diseases such as cardiovascular and respiratory diseases can be reduced drastically by (controlling, promoting, threatening) a low-carbon society.
2. (Nicolas Watts, Maria Neira, Alistair Woodward) says that around two million premature deaths a year will be cut by reducing black carbon emissions.
3. In 2003, approximately 70,000 people in Europe died because of (floods, air pollution, abnormally hot weather).
4. WHO warns that about (250 thousand, 3 million, 1.2 million) people will die every year from the effects of global warming.
5. According to the Lancet Commission report, air pollution is linked to around 1.2 million deaths (in China alone, in Asia, worldwide).

B 音声を聴いて，次の英文の（ ）内に適語を記入しなさい。　track 03～07

1. Climate change causes (　　　)(　　　)(　　　)(　　　) deaths every year.
2. The combustion of fossil fuels produces (　　　)(　　　)(　　　) carbon dioxide emissions.
3. The findings presented by the research group (　　　)(　　　)(　　　) those of the previous study.
4. (　　　)(　　　)(　　　) toxic substances we consume can have adverse effects on the brain.
5. (　　　)(　　　)(　　　) happens, we should complete the task by the appointed date.

C 和文に合うように，（ ）内の語句を並べかえて英文をつくりなさい。

1. 多くの国々が二酸化炭素の排出を半分減らすよう中国に強く促した。
   (China, reduce, by, urged, CO_2 emissions, to, many countries, half).

2. 自然災害による被害は，今年およそ3500億円に達すると見積もられている。
   (about 350 billion yen, to, caused, estimated, this year, reach, by, natural disasters, the damage, is).

3. 健康的なライフスタイルへの移行が，生活の質を高めるために求められている。
   (improve, healthy lifestyle, to, required, a quality of life, to, is, a shift).

4. 地球温暖化が進むにつれ，感染症が拡大するだろう。
   (infectious disease, as, warmer, will, gets, spread, the world).

5. 環境によいと思うことを実行に移すべきである。
   (is, the environment, we, what, for, think, should, good, put in practice, we).

D 次の英語に相当する日本語を下から選び，記号で答えなさい。

1. weather extremes （ ）　　2. agricultural productivity （ ）
3. infectious disease （ ）　　4. air pollution （ ）
5. greenhouse gas （ ）　　6. premature death （ ）
7. renewable energy （ ）　　8. respiratory disease （ ）
9. communicable disease （ ）　　10. cardiovascular disease （ ）

a. 感染症	b. 再生可能エネルギー	c. 循環器系疾患
d. 農業生産性	e. 異常気象	f. 温室効果ガス
g. 呼吸器系疾患	h. 早世	i. 大気汚染
j. 伝染病		

Unit 2

肥満という流行病

Researcher: Obesity Poses Complex Problem
Voice of America, May 25, 2015

track 08

　For the last 15 years, Plymouth, England has held a symposium on obesity. It's estimated that more than half the city's adults are overweight or obese. The rest of Britain is not faring much better. But what's happening in the U.K. can also be seen in the U.S. and many Western countries and a growing number of developing nations. One obesity expert said it's a long term problem that is very difficult to solve.

　Professor Jonathan Pinkney said, "No one health issue has the most impact on human health, or engenders more debate about how to tackle it, than obesity." Pinkney - a professor of Endocrinology and Diabetes – took part in the annual Plymouth Symposium on Obesity, Diabetes and Metabolic Syndrome on May 21.

　He said obesity is a complex issue that involves more than calorie intake.

　"I personally feel that this is such a wide field. There are so many issues. There's politics. There's biology. There's everything you can imagine. There's the food industry. And I think that sometimes we're all a bit guilty of just maybe concentrating on one of those areas. And you can go to a conference anywhere in the world where they spend days just talking about bariatric surgery or fizzy drinks. So, I think it's right to talk about everything under one umbrella."

　Bariatric surgery restricts how much food a person can eat, sharply reducing caloric intake.

　The professor gave his definition of obesity as "when body size becomes so huge that it impairs people's day to day function and quality of life and well-being and personal

Notes:

obesity／(病的な)肥満　Plymouth／プリマス(イングランド南西部の港湾都市)　symposium／シンポジウム　more than ～／～以上の　obese／(病的に)肥満の　the rest of ～／～の残り　fare／やっていく, 暮らす　a growing number of ～／ますます多くの～　have an impact on ～／～に影響を与える　engender／引き起こす　endocrinology／内分泌学　diabetes／糖尿病　take part in ～／～に参加する　metabolic syndrome／代謝(異常)症候群　calorie／カロリー　intake／摂取　biology／生物学　spend A (時間) ～ ing／A (時間)を～することに費やす　bariatric surgery／肥満手術　fizzy drink／炭酸飲料　so ～ that ...／とても～なので…　impair／損なう　day to day／毎日の　quality of life／生活の質　well-being／幸福

relationships. Yeah, that's kind of devastating. That tends to occur at a higher level of body weight."

However, Pinkney said those not considered technically obese are also at high risk for poor health.

"That's the more important point for the health of the population. You know, all the diabetes and heart attacks and cancers and things. I mean that's really caused by lower levels of weight gain. As you can see, it's just the average weight of the population drifting up because we're just sort of eating the wrong things and not really sufficiently active," he said.

The Plymouth symposium showed that much is known about the biology of the brain and appetite control. But Pinkney said, as one speaker pointed out, knowledge is not enough.

"That is completely overridden by things going on around us in the environment: food advertising – food Industry -- the way that it's all marketed to everybody, including children. And I think the simple fact of the matter is, you know, our bodies are very smart and beautifully built. But it's just that the biological systems that would keep us slim are just completely swept away by the pressure from the things going on around us," he said.

And he said it's difficult to do anything about it whether in Britain, the U.S. or developing countries that have adopted a Western diet heavy in sugar, salt and fat.

"There's a multinational food industry and there's huge vested interest in selling a lot of the stuff. I can't give you a magic word as to how you crack this, but we've got exactly the same problem here. And I think you can prescribe all the drugs you want. You can do all the bariatric surgery you could manage to fund, but it's not going to crack the problem unless you stop the development of the epidemic at source," said Pinkney.

Going to the source means how eating habits are formed. Poor eating habits can be a learned behavior passed down by parents to their children.

"I think a lot of things start very early in life. You know, it's difficult to break the habits of a lifetime, isn't it? I think we all find that. But I think our health and our prospects for the future are kind of laid down fairly early. And I think that's not

Notes:

kind of ～／ある程度～　devastating／壊滅的な　tend to ～／～する傾向がある　heart attack／心臓発作　cancer／がん　sort of ～／ある程度～　appetite／食欲　point out ～／～を指摘する　override ～／～に優先する，～より先である　whether A or B／AであろうとBであろうと　multinational／多国籍の　vested interest／既得権益　as to ～／～について　prescribe／処方する　manage to ～／なんとか～する　fund／資金を出す　epidemic／流行病　at source／もとのところで　pass down／代々伝える

surprising. Big kids often have big parents. I think they learn this at an early stage," he said.

Solving the problem, he said, is a lot harder than simply trying to encourage prevention.

55 "There isn't a kind of medical way to prevent the problem. It really does look as if it's down to politics, policy, marketing, food industry and preventing children from being exposed to all of this," Pinkney said. "And I think that's the toughest thing that we face in the world. It's very, very difficult."

Pinkney said too many unrefined carbohydrates – sugars – are to blame for much of 60 the obesity epidemic. He said that they don't satisfy a person's hunger for long and people eat their next meal sooner.

"Commercially produced processed food with large amounts of carbohydrate – sweeteners, short acting carbohydrate – and it just sets us up to fail. And I think there are big problems with carbohydrate in the Western diet," he said.

65 While it may be difficult to foster better eating habits, Pinkney said there is precedent for large scale behavior change.

"Other things have changed. I mean one really interesting thing, I think, was what's happened over cigarette smoking. And how people complained about not being able to smoke in pubs and restaurants and have to go outside. But it didn't take very long for 70 that to translate into clear health benefit. So, you know, maybe you can get these things through in time, little by little," he said.

Some lessons, he said, can be learned from our hunter-gatherer ancestors.

"The hunter-gatherers going right back to last Ice Age and before that would have had a diet that was rich in complex, sort of, fiber kind of carbohydrate. There would be 75 protein in it now and again. But it didn't have all the sugar. So, the diet that is, of course, followed by traditional peoples is radically different."

He said studies of indigenous peoples, who returned to their traditional diets, "took a step back from modern health problems." Pinkney says a combination of prevention methods, medical interventions and political will will be needed to stop the obesity 80 epidemic.

Notes:

as if ～／まるで～であるかのように　be down to ～／～のせいである，～の責任である　prevent A from ～ing／Aが～することを防ぐ　unrefined carbohydrates／精製されていない炭水化物　processed food／加工食品　foster／助長する　precedent／前例　complain about ～／～について不満をいう　translate into ～／～に変わる　get A through／Aをやり終える　in time／そのうちに　little by little／少しずつ　hunter-gatherer／狩猟採集民　be rich in ～／～が豊富である　now and again／ときどき　indigenous／先住の

In the U.S. the Centers for Disease Control and Prevention reported over 35 percent of adults – or nearly 79 million people – are obese. More 17 million children were obese. The annual medical cost of obesity in the U.S. is nearly $200 million.

Notes:
the Centers for Disease Control and Prevention／疾病管理予防センター

練習問題

A 次の英文が，本文の内容と一致する場合にはT，一致しない場合にはFを（ ）内に記入しなさい。

1. （   ） Obesity epidemic cannot be seen in developing countries.
2. （   ） Obesity is a problem of calorie intake.
3. （   ） Obesity damages the quality of life and personal relationships.
4. （   ） There are few problems with carbohydrate in Western food.
5. （   ） We will need a combination of prevention methods, medical intervention and political will to stop the obesity epidemic.

B 音声を聴いて，次の英文の（ ）内に適語を記入しなさい。　track 09〜13

1. (   ) large (   ) (   ) tickets were sold almost immediately.
2. These traditions have been (   ) (   ) from one generation to the next.
3. She behaved (   ) (   ) nothing had happened.
4. Nearly all nuts (   ) (   ) (   ) protein.
5. She comes to Los Angeles every (   ) (   ) (   ).

C 和文に合うように，（ ）内の語句を並べかえて英文をつくりなさい。

1. 最近の事故が原因で，彼女はそのレースに参加することができなかった。
   (the race, part, to, was, her recent accident, she, in, unable, of, take, because).

2. 指導者が変わったことで，政府の方針にも大きな影響があるだろう。
   (government policy, a, will, impact, leadership, on, make, the change, great, in).

3. 私の母は週末の大半を使って家の掃除をした。
   (the house, the weekend, up, spent, of, my mother, cleaning, most).

4. あらゆることがあまりにも変わっていたので，その場所だということがわからなかった。
   (hardly, that, the place, much, I, everything, recognize, changed, so, has, can).

5. 両親は彼がガールフレンドと暮らすために出て行かないようにした。
   (going, with, to, from, live, to, him, his parents, his girlfriend, tried, prevent).

D 次の英語に相当する日本語を下から選び，記号で答えなさい。

1. diabetes （　）　　　2. heart attack （　）
3. cancer （　）　　　4. leukemia （　）
5. hepatitis （　）　　　6. stroke （　）
7. depression （　）　　　8. myocardial infarction （　）
9. tuberculosis （　）　　　10. dementia （　）

a. 心筋梗塞	b. がん	c. 結核
d. うつ病	e. 糖尿病	f. 肝炎
g. 脳卒中	h. 白血病	i. 認知症
j. 心臓発作		

Unit 3
「尊厳死」か「自殺ほう助」か？ ― 米国の終末期医療の側面

In US, Growing Push for 'Aid in Dying' for Terminally Ill
Voice of America, April 9, 2015

 track 14

NEW YORK—

Sara Myers was diagnosed four years ago with amyotrophic lateral sclerosis (ALS), a paralyzing, always fatal neurodegenerative disease.

"At the time I was told three to five years life expectancy. I am traveling down this road, not at a fast pace, but not at a slow pace either," Myers, 60, said recently in her New York apartment, where she is confined to a wheelchair. "I am losing my ability to breathe, and I am opting not to go for a tracheotomy or ventilator."

"I've been trying to live each day as fully as I can," she continued. "But when it gets to the point that my bad days outweigh the good, and I know that it's only going to get worse, then I might decide to end my suffering then."

Myers wants to be able to end her life with a lethal drug dose, if she chooses, while she is still able to swallow. She is among eight patients and medical professionals who filed suit in New York State Supreme Court recently, challenging a state law that bars physicians from prescribing life-ending drugs to dying patients.

"This is really about a patient's choice to determine how he or she is going to die. It's not a question of whether a patient is going to die, it's a question of how they're going to do it, and who's going to make that decision" said David Leven, executive director of

Notes:

be diagnosed with ～／～であると診断される　amyotrophic lateral sclerosis (ALS)／筋萎縮性側索硬化症（きんいしゅくせいそくさくこうかしょう）　paralyzing／麻痺させる，麻痺性の　fatal／致命的な（死が不可避であることを暗示する）　neurodegenerative／神経変性の　life expectancy／平均余命　be confined to ～／～に留め置かれる　opt to ～／選んで～する，～することを決める　go for ～／～を目指す，求める　tracheotomy／気管切開（術）　ventilator／人工呼吸器　outweigh ～／～より勝る　lethal／致死の　dose／（薬の）服用量（の一回分）　file suit／提訴を起こす　New York State Supreme Court／ニューヨーク州最高裁判所(Supreme Court Appellate of New York（高等裁判所）とは別)　bar A from ～ ing／Aが～することを禁止する　physician／医師(狭義の意味で「内科医」)

End of Life Choices New York, another plaintiff in the suit brought by the Disability Rights Legal Center.

Like others in the aid in dying movement, as supporters call it, Leven contends that it should not be considered suicide when a mentally competent adult in the end stages of terminal illness takes a lethal drug. But in all but five U.S. states it is illegal for physicians to assist terminal patients in ending their lives. The exceptions are Oregon, Washington, New Mexico, Montana and Vermont.

A patient's choice

Oregon's "Death with Dignity" law is the best-known, largely because of the recent YouTube advocacy of Brittany Maynard.

A 29-year-old newlywed diagnosed with incurable brain cancer, Maynard did not want to die semiconscious or suffering in a hospital bed. She chose to move from California to Oregon in time to qualify as a resident and receive a lethal prescription.

"I want to be sure my husband and mother are with me when I die. I want to leave this earth in my home, in the arms of my husband and my parents," she said in one of the videos she made before she ended her life last November.

The Oregon law requires two physicians to certify that a patient has a life expectancy of less than six months, is mentally competent, not suffering from depression, and is not being coerced. Patients must make two requests for aid in dying separated by 15 days, as well as a written, witnessed request, and must take the medication themselves.

In the 18 years since the law took effect, 1,173 people have received such prescriptions and 752 have ended their lives with them, according to state statistics

---

Notes:

End of Life Choices New York／（EOLCNY）ニューヨーク市に本部を置く団体。ホスピス，延命治療等，カウンセリングや訴訟にも対応し，個々の終末期に関する選択のためのサービスを提供する　plaintiff／原告　Disability Rights Legal Center／米国ロサンゼルスに本部を置く障害者権利のための団体。障害をもつ個人の意志による終末期選択を法的に解決する　the aid in dying movement／米国における終末期援助に対して，法改正も含め積極的にかかわろうとする一連の運動　contend／主張する　mentally competent／精神的能力のある　all but ～／～を除いてすべて　terminal patients／終末期患者　Death with Dignity／尊厳死　because of ～／～が理由で　advocacy／主張，提唱　incurable／不治の　semiconscious／半覚醒の，半ば意識が朦朧とした　in time to ～／～するのに間に合って　qualify as ～／～としての資格を得る　lethal／致死の　prescription／処方箋　certify ～／～を証明する　suffer from ～／～に苦しむ，～を病む　depression／鬱　be coerced／強要された　A as well as B／BだけでなくAも　take (the) medication／薬剤投与を受ける　take effect／効力を生ずる　according to ～／～によれば　statistics／統計（複数扱い）

quoted in a report by Compassion & Choices, a group that advocates for laws like Oregon's. The group says that simply having the medicine as an option creates peace of mind for some dying people, who then choose to let the disease take its course.

Since Maynard's death, lawmakers in at least 20 states, including New York and California, have introduced bills to legalize physician-assisted dying. They are opposed on religious grounds by Roman Catholic leaders, as well as by some disability rights groups who say the laws will be abused and lead to euthanasia.

Under pressure

T.K. Small, of the group Not Dead Yet, says patients will be pressured to end their lives, because health care for the dying is very costly, while lethal drugs are cheap.

"When you have a $300 prescription, versus a very expensive chemotherapy regime or just having somebody to help you in your home, that's expensive," he said in an interview. "A person who is a caregiver, who stands to inherit money, can be a witness when these forms and prescriptions are requested from a doctor. An individual receiving money under a will can literally go pick up the medicine, and there's no other witnesses [to the death] involved."

Small noted that the terminally ill are able to speed up death by refusing food and fluids, while accepting pain medication. He would choose that palliative care method, he said.

"From what I hear there's more morphine than you can shake a stick at in these palliative-care practices. It wouldn't take long, a few days," he said, adding, "I would feel comfortable knowing that I hadn't compromised the existences of other people."

Aid-in-dying proponents maintain that the palliative option can still entail great suffering, and isn't ethically different from timing one's death via a drug. Some people, bedridden and retaining fluid, have lived as long as two weeks. In her final video,

---

Notes:

quote／引用する　Compassion & Choices／コロラド州デンバーにあるNPOで，終末期の選択肢について提言を行っている　take one's course／（病気が）自然の経過をたどる　lawmaker／立法者，議員　at least／少なくとも　bill／法案　oppose／反対する　on religious ground／宗教的な理由で　abuse／悪用する，乱用する　euthanasia／安楽死　Not Dead Yet（NDY）／「まだ死んではいない」米国にある障害者の権利のための団体で，自殺ほう助や安楽死に反対している　the dying／死に逝く者　versus ～／～に対比して，比較して　chemotherapy regime／化学療法計画（regimeはregimenと同義）　caregiver／介護者　stand to ～／～しそうである　inherit／（財産，遺産などを）相続する　palliative care／緩和ケア　more ～ than one can shake a stick at／通常よりも～が多いことがわかる（shake a stick at～「～に気づく」）　morphine／モルヒネ　compromise／（信用などを）傷つける　entail／必然的に伴う　timing／時期を選ぶこと　retain／維持する　as long as ～／～ものあいだ

Brittany Maynard explained why she had rejected palliative care.

"I can't imagine what that experience would be like. I may be minimally conscious, still suffering and unable to move or speak," she said, adding, "Death with dignity is a much swifter and peaceful way to pass."

Supporters also contend that legalizing physician-prescribed aid in dying will prevent premature, often violent suicides by people diagnosed with terminal illness. Marcia Angell, a former editor of *the New England Journal of Medicine*, has written that her father, who shot himself rather than endure a lingering death from metastatic cancer, might have chosen to live longer had he known he could ingest a drug that would enable him to die quickly and without pain. In an essay for *the New York Review of Books*, she asked, "Why should anyone - the state, the medical profession, or anyone else - presume to tell someone else how much suffering they must endure as their life is ending?"

Recent polls report that a majority of Americans are coming to agree: about three out of four Americans now believe that terminally ill patients in pain should have the right to end their lives. A majority of physicians and several medical associations also now support legalizing physician-assisted deaths. The American Medical Association, however, continues to oppose legalization, saying it is "fundamentally incompatible with the physician's role as healer, would be difficult or impossible to control, and would pose societal risks."

Notes:

premature／早まった　*the New England Journal of Medicine*／ニューイングランド・ジャーナル・オブ・メディシン。マサチューセッツ内科外科医学会が刊行する英文の総合医学雑誌　A rather than B／BよりもむしろA　endure／耐え忍ぶ　lingering／ぐずぐず長引く　metastatic cancer／転移性腫瘍　had he known ～／～を知っていたなら（＝if he had known ～）　ingest／（薬などを）摂取する　enable A to ～／Aが～できるようにする　presume to (do)／おこがましくも～する　poll／世論調査　three out of four／4（人）のうちの3（人）　the American Medical Association／米国医師会　incompatible with ～／～と相容れない　societal／（socialと同義）

練習問題

A 次の英文が，本文の内容と一致する場合にはT，一致しない場合にはFを（　）内に記入しなさい。

1. (　) Sara Myers had to drive at not a fast pace because she developed ALS.
2. (　) It is legal in Montana State that doctors prescribe terminal illness patients a lethal drug.
3. (　) It has been more than twenty years since the law of "Death with Dignity" was put into operation in the State of Oregon.
4. (　) Mr. Small insists that any legal heir could be a supporter of the aid in dying movement.
5. (　) The American Medical Association has been against physician-prescribed aid in dying because doctors cannot control the law.

B 音声を聴いて，次の英文の（　）内に適語を記入しなさい。　track 15〜19

1. He (　　　) (　　　) go alone.
2. Nothing (　　　) him (　　　) leaving his office.
3. His desires (　　　) (　　　) (　　　) his income.
4. Nearly (　　　) (　　　) (　　　) (　　　) Americans is considered obese.
5. The actress (　　　) (　　　) (　　　) hepatitis B.

C 和文に合うように，（　）内の語句を並べかえて英文をつくりなさい。

1. なるように任せなさい（打っちゃっておけ）
   (their, things, take, own, leave, to, course).

2. 彼女がもしその億万長者の娘だと証明されれば，金持ちになりそうだ。
   She (proven, stands, if, to, to, become, be, she, is, a daughter, the billionaire, rich, of).

Unit 3　17

3. この辺りには本当にホームレスの人たちがいっぱいだ。
　 (people, this neighborhood, homeless, you, shake, has, a stick, can, than, at, more).

4. その夜，3人を除き私のクラスの全員が，先生の開いたパーティーに顔を見せた。
　 (my, students, three, teacher's, night, showed, all, in, up, our, party, but, to, that, class).

5. その法律が効力を生じるようになってから，多くのタイ人が査証免除で訪日している。
　 (many, without, visa, Thai, effect, visited, the law, since, have, took, Japan).

D 次の英語に相当する日本語を下から選び，記号で答えなさい。

1. neurological system　　（　）系　　2. cardiovascular system　（　）系
3. respiratory system　　　（　）系　　4. digestive system　　　　（　）系
5. endocrine system　　　　（　）系　　6. urologic system　　　　　（　）系
7. sensory system　　　　　（　）系　　8. reproductive system　　（　）系
9. musculoskeletal system　（　）系

a. 神経	b. 呼吸器	c. 泌尿器
d. 生殖器	e. 内分泌	f. 循環器
g. 知覚器	h. 筋骨格	i. 消化器

Unit 4
医療現場におけるロボット活躍の可能性

Robot Helps Heal Human Muscle Damage
Voice of America, September 18, 2015

 track 20

Recovering strength and movement after an injury often involves physical therapy. Physical therapists help patients with brain or bone injuries regain control of their muscles. Exercising muscles is an important part of the rehabilitation process. Therapists use balls and boards to improve balance, stretchy bands to increase strength and other exercises.

But a Polish technology company Egzotech has developed a robot called Luna, to make those exercises interactive. Luna can help therapists choose the best exercises for their patients. The robot also provides therapists with information about their patients' progress.

Luna uses electromyography, or EMG, to identify electrical currents as patients bend their arms or legs. Michal Mikulski is the chief executive officer of Egzotech. He says detecting muscle tension not immediately visible to the human eye can help therapists design better exercises.

"We reach a certain stage of disease development…when the muscle tension is not even visible. But these signals can still be seen on our machines. Luna is still able to detect them. And based on that, when the brain sends a signal to the muscle to flex,

---

Notes:

recover／取り戻す　injury／怪我　involve／含む　physical therapy／理学療法　physical therapist／理学療法士　help A ～／Aが～するのを手助けする　regain／取り戻す　rehabilitation process／リハビリの経過　board／板　improve／改善する　stretchy band／伸縮性バンド（運動するためのゴム製伸縮帯）　increase／増強する　Polish／ポーランドの　Egzotech／エグゾテック（ポーランドの企業で，おもにリハビリの際に利用される外骨格を製造販売）　develop／開発する　interactive／相互作用のある，体験型の　provide A with B／AにBを提供する　progress／経過　electromyography: EMG／筋電位（筋肉を動かすときに生じる電圧）　identify／確認する　electrical current／電流　bend／曲げる　the chief executive officer／最高経営責任者　detect／検出する，感知する　muscle tension／筋張力（筋が収縮しようとする力）　immediately／すぐに　visible to ～／～に見える　reach a certain stage／ある段階に到達する　disease development／病気の進行　signal／兆候　based on that／それに基づいて　flex／曲げる

even though we don't see it, Luna is still able to detect it. It detects these signals and causes the movement of the limb, as if it were performed naturally."

Luna can also make therapy fun for children who often get bored with repeated movements. Luna permits them to play games without knowing that they are exercising their muscles.

"Sometimes it is a spacecraft, sometimes shooting balls, sometimes flying a dragon. In any case, a child wants to win a game, wants to compete, but in fact they are exercising."

Luna is just a prototype. But Egzotech expects to have other robots ready for sale later this year.

Robot Scientist Helps Design New Drugs
Voice of America, September 18 2015

 track 21

Robots are common in today's world. They manufacture cars, work in space, explore oceans, clean up oil spills and investigate dangerous environments. And now, scientists at the University of Manchester are using a robot as a laboratory partner.

The researchers at the university created the robot in 2009 and named it Adam. Despite the name, Adam is not a humanoid robot. It is about the size of a car.

Adam was built to do science and make discoveries. Ross King is the leader of the University of Manchester research team. He says the robot made a discovery about yeast, a kind of fungus used in science as a model for human cells.

"Adam hypothesized certain functions of genes within yeast and experimentally tested these hypothesizes and confirmed them. So it both hypothesized and confirmed new scientific knowledge."

Notes:
even though ~／たとえ～でも　cause／引き起こす　limb／手足　as if ~／あたかも～であるかのように　perform／行う　get bored with ~／～に退屈する　repeated／繰り返される　permit A to ~／Aに～することを許可する　without knowing that ~／～であることに気づかないうちに　spacecraft／宇宙船　in any case／いずれにせよ　compete／競争する　in fact／実際は　prototype／試作品　expect to ~／～すると期待する　have other robots ready／have A B でAをBの状態に保っておく　(be) ready for ~／～の準備を整える　manufacture／製造する　explore／調査する　oil spill／油流出　investigate／調査する　laboratory／実験　despite ~／～にもかかわらず　humanoid robot／人型ロボット　make a discovery／発見する　yeast／イースト菌　fungus／菌類　cell／細胞　hypothesize／仮定・仮定する　functions of a gene／遺伝子機能　experimentally／実験的に　confirm／（正しいと）確認する

Adam's success as a scientist led to the creation of another robot scientist named Eve. Researchers developed Eve to design and test drugs for tropical and neglected diseases. These diseases kill and infect millions of people each year.

Drug development is slow and costly. Experts say it can take more than 10 years and about $1 billion to discover and develop new medicines. Drug manufacturers are unlikely to get their investment money back.

So the University of Manchester developed a low-cost test that shows whether or not a chemical is likely to be made into an effective medicine. Mr. King says that other drug testing methods were not very effective.

"How it works conventionally is you use robotics as well and you have a large collection of possible drugs. You test every single compound. And you start at the beginning of your library and continue until the end, and stop. So it's not a very intelligent process. The robotics doesn't learn anything as it goes along, even if it's tested a million compounds, it still doesn't have any expectation of what will happen next when it tests a new compound."

Mr. King says that Eve is different because the robot learns as it tests different compounds. He says the robot is designed to ignore compounds that it thinks unlikely to be good. It will only test the compounds which have a good chance of working.

Eve has discovered that a compound known to be effective against cancer might also be used to fight against malaria and other tropical diseases.

Mr. King says he hopes to completely automate the drug testing process with robots like Eve to create and test new chemicals. But he says humans remain in control of the manufacturing process.

Notes:

lead to ～／～につながる　creation／創造　tropical／熱帯性の　neglected／放置された, 無視された　infect／伝染する　millions of ～／何百万もの～　development／開発　costly／費用のかかる　expert／専門家　it takes（時間）and（金額）to ～／～するのに（時間）と（金額）がかかる　more than ～／～以上の　manufacturer／製造メーカー　be unlikely to ～／～しそうにない　investment money／投資資金　low-cost／費用のかからない　whether or not ～／～かどうか　chemical／化学物質　be likely to ～／～しそうである　effective／効果のある　conventionally／従来, 伝統的に, 通常　robotics／ロボット工学　have a large collection of ～／～をたくさん集めている　every single／ありとあらゆる　compound／化合物　library／遺伝子や化合物の網羅的コレクション　intelligent／賢明な　as it goes along／進むにつれて　even if it's tested ～／たとえそれが～をテストしたとしても（＝even if it has tested ～）　expectation／予想　be designed to ～／～するように設計されている　ignore／無視する　good chance of ～ing／～する十分な可能性　known to ～／～であると知られている　effective against ～／～に対して効果がある　fight against ～／～に対して抵抗する　malaria／マラリア　completely／完全に　automate／自動化する　remain ～／～のままでいる　in control of ～／～を制御して　the manufacturing process／製造過程

Damaged Robots Learn to Make Changes to Keep Working

Voice of America, September 18, 2015

track 22

When a dog loses a leg, the animal eventually figures out the best way to get around on three legs. In a short time, the dog learns to deal with its physical disability.

Now, scientists have developed robots that behave in much the same way.

We can find robots everywhere. Robots build cars, play chess and can clean your house. They may someday drive your car, too.

Two robots, named Spirit and Opportunity, were sent to Mars on a mission to explore the red planet.

Jeff Clune is a computer scientist with the University of Wyoming. He says robots also help people in natural disasters.

Robots are deployed in search and rescue operations following an earthquake. They may someday also be used to examine the wreckage of a nuclear accident, like the one in Fukushima, Japan.

Mr. Clune says robots can be sent to a lot of places said to be unsafe.

"The problem is that all of those types of situations and environment are extremely unpredictable and hostile. And it is very likely that robots and humans in those situations become damaged."

He and other scientists are developing technology so that robots will continue operating after the first sign of injury. They want the machines to have the ability to make changes and continue performing until they can be repaired.

Mr. Clune and researchers in France have added one more operation to the skill set of robots working under difficult conditions. They say they programmed a hexapod robot, one with six legs, and a robotic arm to learn how to deal with injury. Their findings were reported in the journal "Nature."

Notes:

eventually／やがては　figure out／わかる　get around／歩き回る　in a short time／まもなく　deal with ～／～に対処する　physical disability／身体的不能　named ～／～と名付けられた　on a mission to ～／～する目的で　natural disaster／自然災害　deploy／配備する　search and rescue／捜索救助，救難　operation／作業　following ～／～の後の　earthquake／地震　examine／調べる　wreckage／残骸　nuclear accident／原子力事故　said to be ～／～といわれている　extremely／極度に　unpredictable／想定外の，予想できない　hostile／好ましくない　it is likely that ～／おそらく～であろう　become damaged／損害を受ける　so that S will ～／Sが～できるように　want A to ～／Aに～してほしい　the ability to ～／～する能力　repair／修理する　hexapod robot／六脚のロボット　finding／発見

Mr. Clune said that once the robots become damaged, they use their intuition and
25　knowledge of how their body works to find a way to deal with the damage.

He says the robots are also programmed with child-like curiosity. In other words, they are always asking questions and looking for answers. The whole process takes about a minute for the robots to find a way to overcome damage.

Notes:

once ～／いったん～すると　intuition／直感　child-like／子供のような　curiosity／好奇心　in other words／いい換えれば　look for ～／～を求める　take ～ for A to ...／Aが…するのに～かかる　overcome／乗り越える

練 習 問 題

A 本文の内容に合うように，各英文の（　）内に入る最も適切な語句をそれぞれ1つずつ選びなさい。

1. The Robot Luna, provides therapists with information about (their patients' disease / their patients' injury / their patients' progress).
2. The Robot Luna, can make therapy (fun / hard / easy) for children who often get bored with repeated movements.
3. The robot, Eve, was developed to design and test drugs for (cancers / tropical diseases / injuries).
4. The University of Manchester developed (an expensive / an inexpensive / a difficult) test to show if a chemical can be made into an effective medicine.
5. The hexapod robot was programmed to learn (how to deal with injury / how to build cars / how to play chess).

B 音声を聴いて，次の英文の（　）内に適語を記入しなさい。　track 23～27

1. He behaves (　　　) (　　　) he were my old friend.
2. She went to see her boss to confirm (　　　) (　　　) (　　　) she had to go with him.
3. He has been (　　　) (　　　) (　　　) that section for a long time.
4. I can't (　　　) (　　　) the cause of the accident at all.
5. My grandmother cannot hear me well, (　　　) (　　　) (　　　), she is slightly deaf.

C 和文に合うように，（　）内の語句を並べかえて英文をつくりなさい。

1. 図書館で私が本を探すのを手伝ってくれるなんて，彼女は親切だった。
   (look for, the library, kind, was, me, a book, at, she, to, help).

2. 時間を無駄にしていることも知らずに，子どもたちはコンピューターゲームに夢中になった。
   (knowing, the computer game, the children, in, without, wasted, were absorbed, that, time, it).

3. この仕事を終えるのに8カ月かかった。
   (months, this work, it, eight, to, took, complete).

4. 勇気があるといわれている兵士たちが城の周りにたくさんいた。
   (brave, were, said, the castle, many, there, soldiers, to, around, be).

5. その教師は，クラスの生徒たちみんなに試験に合格してほしかった。
   (the students, the exam, the teacher, to, wanted, pass, all, in the class).

D 次の英語に相当する日本語を下から選び，記号で答えなさい。

1. stretchy band　　　（　）
2. electromyography　（　）
3. muscle tension　　（　）
4. limb　　　　　　　（　）
5. fungus　　　　　　（　）
6. cell　　　　　　　（　）
7. functions of genes（　）
8. infect　　　　　　（　）
9. chemical　　　　　（　）
10. compound　　　　　（　）

a. 手足　　　　b. 細胞　　　　c. 遺伝子機能
d. 菌類　　　　e. 化学物質　　f. 化合物
g. 筋電位　　　h. 筋張力　　　i 伸縮性バンド
j. 伝染する

Unit 5

産科フィスチュラ撲滅をめざして

UN Report Links Progress with Efforts to End Fistula
Voice of America, August 21, 2015

track 28

The final Millennium Development Goals report on maternal mortality for middle- and low-income countries was recently released. It says many countries around the world have reduced maternal mortality by nearly half, which is great progress.

However, the global women's health organization EngenderHealth Inc. says the world must not overlook the impact of maternal injuries, such as obstetric fistula, on the life of a mother. The group says fistula ruins a woman's chances of having a livelihood, raising a healthy family and contributing to her community. And it argues that eliminating fistula means eradicating obstructed labor.

Obstetric Fistula results when obstructed labor causes a hole between the birth canal and the bladder or rectum. It leaves women leaking urine, feces or both, and over time, it leads to chronic medical problems.

According to the report, the still-high rate of obstetric fistula means much work still needs to be done in addressing maternal healthcare.

Dr. Lauri Romanzi, is the project director for Fistula Care Plus, a project of EngenderHealth, Inc. The project is funded by the U.S. Agency for International Development, (USAID). She says obstetric fistula is part of a long list of deadly problems caused by obstructed labor.

"The relationship between fistula and maternal mortality is simply that obstructed

Notes:

fistula ／（産科）瘻孔，フィスチュラ　Millennium Development Goals ／ミレニアム開発目標(MDGs)　maternal mortality (rate) ／妊産婦死亡(率)　release ／公表する　overlook ／見落とす　such as ～／～のような　obstetric ／産科の　ruin ／だめにする，台なしにする　livelihood ／生活手段，生計　contribute to ～／～に貢献する　argue ／主張する　eradicate ／根絶する　obstructed labor ／閉塞性分娩，分娩停止　birth canal ／産道　bladder ／膀胱　rectum ／直腸　leave A ～ing ／Aを～のままにする　urine ／尿　feces ／大便　over time ／徐々に　lead to ～／～につながる　chronic ／慢性の　medical problem ／内科的疾患　according to ～／～によれば　still-high ／依然として高い　address ／（困難な状況などに）立ち向かう，取り組む　U.S. Agency for International Development (USAID) ／アメリカ合衆国国際開発庁

labor often kills women. But if it does not kill the woman, then she will have any number of morbidities, only one of which is obstetric fistula. She can also have severe internal scarring that make sexual relations impossible. She can have infertility, nerve damage that makes it impossible to walk properly," said Romanzi.

"A lot of women," she said, "have what is in essence post-traumatic stress disorder. They're mourning very often the loss of a stillborn baby. They have anxiety, depression, difficulty concentrating and this can persist even after they have been treated for the fistula condition, and successfully so."

Romanzi emphasized that fistula ruins a woman's life because she is perpetually incontinent of either feces, urine or both.

"Here in the U.S., incontinence is either the number one or number two reason to admit someone to a nursing home," she said. "There's no human community anywhere in the world that finds living with a constantly incontinent person to be something that is easily tolerated."

In contrast, she said, "in poor countries women who have become constantly incontinent as a result of fistula don't have the option of being warehoused into a community, so they're often simply ostracized by their community. About 40 to 50 percent of them are divorced. What I find remarkable about that statistic is that we've got about half of the husbands not divorcing their wives. And I think those men deserve to be acknowledged and applauded for continuing to support the mother of their children."

Another consequence of obstructed labor that receives little to no attention is that 70-80 percent of the babies are stillborn. Those who do survive the obstructed birth are born with a condition called hypoxia, or low-oxygen level.

Romanzi pointed out it can take a mother with obstructed labor up to nine days to deliver, which means the baby did not receive adequate oxygen during this period.

Notes:

any number of 〜／いくらでも多くの〜　morbidity／罹患(率)，病的状態　internal scar／体内瘢痕(はんこん)　infertility／不妊(症)　in essence／本質的には，本当は　post-traumatic stress disorder／心的外傷後ストレス障害(PTSD)　mourn／悲しむ，嘆く　stillborn／死産の　anxiety／不安　depression／うつ病，抑うつ症　persist／(好ましくない状況などが)持続する　perpetually／絶え間なく　incontinence／失禁　admit／(病院・施設などに)入院させる，収容する　nursing home／老人ホーム　tolerate／寛大に取り扱う　in contrast／対照的に　as a result of 〜／〜の結果として　option／選択肢　warehouse／収容する　ostracize／排斥する，のけものにする　remarkable／注目に値する　deserve to 〜／〜する価値がある，〜して当然だ　acknowledge／認める　applaud／賞賛する，支持する　those who 〜／〜な人々(この文脈では「生き延びた乳児」をさす)　hypoxia／低酸素症　point out／指摘する　up to 〜／(最高で)〜まで

"These babies are often born paraplegic or quadriplegic, or with severe cerebral palsy, and or with severe intellectual developmental deficits," she said.

Romanzi identified two groups of women who develop fistula in terms of obstetric indicators. The larger of the two groups are mature women who have given birth four or five times previously, and for whatever reason during the mother's next labor, the baby does not come out easily. It is stuck.

"There are many reasons for this. She could have some untreated, undiagnosed gestational diabetes making the baby quite large. She might have a twin pregnancy this time. That's more common as women get older," Romanzi said. "Also, newborn weight tends to be a little larger with each subsequent pregnancy. As women get past the mark of having had five babies, the babies are also more prone to be in a strange position, what's called transverse lie where the baby is sideways. This could lead to obstructed labor."

Another group of women develop fistula with their first baby, even though the young mother may have waited until her late teens or early twenties to have a baby.

"There is this what I call the poster child of fistula—the 12-year-old child bride who gets pregnant before she has her first menses and has an obstructed labor while she's still a small child, possibly with stunted growth due to poor nutrition. And while that's true, that group that gets all the attention in the lay press, is actually a very small component of the total group of women who actually survive obstructed labor and come in with a fistula," said Romanzi.

The main message to learn from these mothers' experiences emphasized Romanzi is that if we want to eradicate obstetric fistula, we must eradicate obstructed labor. Equally important she notes is there is no safe way to give birth without having a skilled birth attendant such as a midwife or doctor, or being at a proper medical center.

"This is something that is missing from a lot of literature. You read that people feel very sorry for these poor women and all the tragedy they face. They want to act like it is

---

Notes:

paraplegic／対麻痺の　quadriplegic／四肢麻痺の　cerebral palsy／脳性麻痺　intellectual developmental deficits／知的発達障害　identify／確認する，気づく　in terms of ～／～の観点から　give birth／出産する　for whatever reason／どんな理由であれ　gestational diabetes／妊娠糖尿病　tend to ～／～する傾向がある　subsequent／あとに続く　be prone to ～／～する傾向がある　transverse lie／横位姿勢　sideways／横に，斜めに　even though ～／～ではあるが　late teens／10代後半　poster child／（病気などを救済する宣伝ポスターに使われる）障害のある子ども，典型的な人物　first menses／初潮　stunted／生育不全の　due to ～／～が原因で　lay press／（新聞などの）マスメディア　component／構成要素　midwife／助産師　literature／文献，論文　like it is something that happens over there／どこかよそで起こっていることのように

something that happens over there when in actuality obstructive labor happens every day everywhere," said Romanzi.

She added, "in high-income countries it is a significant contributor to a cesarean section rate."

EngenderHealth has been working for decades to improve health systems and reproductive health systems for both women and men. Romanzi said access to reliable contraception is the key to reducing the risk of fistula.

"EngenderHealth was originally founded some decades ago with the sole purpose of improving access to family planning and birth-control methods," she said. "As it expanded globally, this remained a core component and wherever we are working with women suffering fistula and fistula Problems. We are also working to make sure that family planning services are available and the delivery mechanism is executed to a global standard."

EngenderHealth also has offered gender equity improvement programs that include men as partners. The programs help men understand what women go through when they are in labor. They learn to recognize danger signs so they can mobilize the mother to get medical care as soon as possible, despite some traditional and cultural beliefs that only strong women have their babies at home.

Notes:

contributor／誘因　cesarean section／帝王切開　decade／10年間　reproductive health／性と生殖に関する健康　access／入手方法　reliable／信頼できる，確実な　contraception／避妊法　with the purpose of ～ing／～という目的で　sole／唯一の　birth-control method／避妊方法　remain／相変わらず～のままである　make sure that ～／必ず～であるように　execute／実行する,実施する　gender equity／男女平等　go through ～／（苦しみなどを）経験する　so S can ～／Sが～できるように　despite ～／～にもかかわらず

練習問題

A 次の英文が，本文の内容と一致する場合にはT，一致しない場合にはFを（ ）内に記入しなさい。

1. （　） According to the final Millennium Development Goals report, many countries have greatly increased maternal mortality.
2. （　） Fistula ruins a woman's life because she is perpetually incontinent of feces and/or urine.
3. （　） One consequence of obstructed labor, 70-80 percent of the babies are stillborn.
4. （　） If we want to eradicate obstetric fistula, we need to develop new vaccines.
5. （　） According to Dr. Romanzi, access to reliable contraception is the key to reducing the risk of getting pregnant.

B 音声を聴いて，次の英文の（ ）内に適語を記入しなさい。　　track 29〜33

1. This library has （　　　）（　　　）（　　　） books, journals and periodicals for the students and faculty.
2. The story may be true （　　　）（　　　） but not necessarily in all details.
3. Rogan had to have surgery （　　　） a （　　　）（　　　） the car accident yesterday.
4. If you want to lose weight （　　　）（　　　）（　　　）, you should take action right now.
5. All passengers should check in （　　　）（　　　） two hours prior to departure of your flight.

C 和文に合うように，（ ）内の語句を並べかえて英文をつくりなさい。

1. 友情が愛情につながることに賛成ですか。
   (agree, love, leads, you, that, do, friendship, to)?

2. あれだけがんばって仕事をしたのだから，マイリーは休暇をとって当然だ。
   (take, Miley, a vacation, deserves, after, hard work, all, that, did, she, to).

3. 食物に含まれる熱量はカロリーで計る。
   (calories, in food, in, of, contained, the amount, of, measured, terms, is, energy).

4. 自分のパスポートを必ず常に携行してください。
   (make, your passport, bring, always, you, please, sure, to, with).

5. 母は腫瘍を摘出する難しい手術を受けた。
   (went, my mother, a, surgery, through, the tumor, difficult, remove, to).

D 次の英語に相当する日本語を下から選び，記号で答えなさい。

1. uterus   ( )   2. birth canal   ( )
3. rectum   ( )   4. colon   ( )
5. bladder   ( )   6. intestines   ( )
7. liver   ( )   8. kidney   ( )
9. stomach   ( ) 10. pancreas   ( )

a. 産道	b. 膀胱	c. 膵臓
d. 腎臓	e. 肝臓	f. 腸
g. 直腸	h. 胃	i. 子宮
j. 結腸		

Unit 6

断食が心身にもたらす効用

Jeanette Winterson: Why I Fasted for 11 Days

The Guardian, July 11, 2015

track 34

The clinic was set up in 1953 by Otto Buchinger, a German doctor who had been discharged from the Imperial German Navy in 1919 with chronic rheumatism of the joints caused by septicaemia. Unable to move without agonising pain, a life in a wheelchair awaited him. He decided to fast for a month and emerged utterly weak but fully mobile. For the rest of his life, into his 80s, he researched the fasting principle.

So what happens when we stop eating? The body first uses up the glycogen stores in the liver. That might take 12 hours, or 24 hours. Afterwards, the body will have to use proteins (muscles) or lipids (fats) to produce the energy (glucose) it needs. The body is programmed to avoid breaking down muscle, and so the liver turns into a factory to manufacture ketones for fuel. That's where all those hokum diets with raspberries and ketone pills come from. But you don't need to buy anything; just stop eating and your body will do the work for you.

This is where the process gets exciting. Imagine your house is freezing and you have to burn the furniture to keep warm. First you burn the rubbish, stuff you have been hoarding for years and don't really need. The body does the same. Sick cells, old cells, decomposed tissues, are burned away. This is the ultimate spring clean. It allows the body to eliminate toxins and metabolic waste at the same time as turning them into

Notes:

Jeanette Winterson／1959年生まれのイギリスの小説家。いくつかの文学賞を受賞しており、その1つで処女作 *Oranges Are Not the Only Fruit* (1985)を始め、日本語訳された作品もある。　be set up ～／～設立される　be discharged from ～／～を除隊になる　the Imperial German Navy／ドイツ帝国海軍　chronic／慢性の　rheumatism／リウマチ　joint／関節　septicaemia／敗血症　agonising pain／苦痛を伴う痛み　emerge utterly weak but fully mobile／(その結果)すっかり体は弱まったが、完全に動けるようになった　use up ～／～を使い果たす　the glycogen stores in the liver／肝臓に貯蔵されているグリコーゲン(storesは、この意味ではしばしば複数形)　lipid／脂質　glucose／ブドウ糖　break down ～／～を(化学的に)分解する　ketone／ケトン(体内のブドウ糖が枯渇して脂肪が分解されるときに、糖に代わる代替エネルギーとして肝臓でつくられる物質)　That's where A comes from.／それがAのそもそもの始まりである　hokum diet／いんちき・まやかしのダイエット　rubbish／がらくた、くず　hoard ～／～を大量にため込む　decomposed tissue／腐敗した組織　ultimate／究極の　spring clean／春の大掃除　toxin／毒素　metabolic waste／代謝老廃物　at the same time as doing ～／～すると同時に

heat and energy. And you can live off this rubbish for days.

Next, the body will go for its fat reserves. Most of us have plenty of fat for the body to get busy on – and belly fat is an easy target. As one doctor at the clinic told me: "You haven't stopped eating – only you are eating from the inside for now."

But the process of ketosis is more than the body eating itself. While fasting, the body goes into repair mode. Valter Longo, professor of Gerontology at the University of Southern California, believes that this protective repairing mechanism is the result of our 3m years of evolution. His ongoing research shows that fasting actively reboots the immune system and leads to a drop in IGF-1, a growth hormone linked to ageing, insulin resistance and tumour progression. There is an impressive documentary available on YouTube called The Science of Fasting. It begins with research carried out over 50 years in the Soviet Union, and until recently unavailable in the west. There, doctors discovered that fasting could successfully treat chronic asthma with a cure rate pharmaceuticals would kill for.

But that's the problem: fasting is free. Well, it's not free, because you need to be medically supervised, at least to begin with, but there's no money in it for Big Pharma. As Dr Andreas Michalsen from the Charité hospital, Berlin – Europe's largest public hospital, and one that treats more than 500 patients a year with fasting – explains in The Science of Fasting: "If I had been studying a new drug and got these results, I would be getting phone calls every day. It is very easy for critics to say there are not enough studies when we know there is no funding for these studies."

* * *

So how do you feel when you fast – you, the person used to having a good relationship with a full fridge?

Notes:

live off ～／～を食べて生きる，～に頼って生きる　go for ～／～を襲う　its fat reserves／体に蓄えた脂肪　plenty of ～／たくさんの～　easy target／(口語)ねらわれやすいもの，いいカモ　ketosis／ケトン症(血中のケトンが異常に増加した状態)　Gerontology／老年学　3m years of revolution／300万年の進化(3m＝3 million)　ongoing／進行中の　reboot the immune system／免疫系を再起動する　growth hormone／成長ホルモン　ageing／老化(＝ aging)　insulin resistance／インシュリン抵抗性(インシュリンに対する感受性が低下し，血糖レベルを調節するインシュリンの作用が十分発揮できない状態)　tumor progression／腫瘍の進行　available／手に入れることができる，利用できる　carry out ～／～を行なう　chronic asthma／慢性喘息　cure rate／治癒率　pharmaceutical／大手製薬会社　would kill for ～／(口語)～のためなら何でもする　be medically supervised／医療的に管理される　at least／少なくとも　to begin with／はじめは　Big Pharma／(＝ big pharmaceutical company, ここでは皮肉を込めた大手製薬会社のよび方)　critic／批判する人　funding／支援財源

The first three days are difficult. Emotionally and physically. The Buchinger method encourages you to accept the mood swings and create an attitude of acceptance and tolerance in yourself; you are working with your body not against it. In the early mornings patients meditate. Exercise classes begin at 8am and run through the day, including long walks and personal training in the gym. Exercise is as important as mindfulness. It keeps the metabolic rate high and encourages the body to move towards a state of maximum efficiency. After all, when we were coping with food shortages in the past, we had to keep moving to find something to eat. Sitting in your room feeling terrible is not the answer.

It helps if you know you are in safe hands. On arrival at Buchinger, patients are given a full set of blood tests and a consultation with a doctor, and every morning a nurse checks your blood pressure and general health. Day three is crisis day as the body moves into full ketone production. I felt cold, withdrawn and a little light-headed. But day four was a revelation: I woke early, clear-eyed, cheerful and full of energy. This continued right through my fast. I was able to concentrate, take long walks and go to the gym. I wasn't hungry for the next six days. My blood pressure was stable throughout, and I was enjoying myself. When the time came to break the fast – something that has to be done most carefully with tiny amounts of solid food – I really wanted to continue, just to see what would happen next.

When my cholesterol was measured it was down from 7.9 to 6.2, and with the "good" cholesterol in the right ratio. Three months later it is stable. Cortisol is back in the normal range. Joint pain in my foot following an operation last year has disappeared completely. If you have weight to lose, you will lose it. If you have less weight to lose, the body seems to know how to balance itself there too.

Fasting isn't a diet. It isn't calorie restriction. After fasting you will return to eating normally, though with adjustments where necessary. But the idea is that while you fast

Notes:

the mood swings／気分の浮き沈み　an attitude of acceptance and tolerance／受容と寛容の心構え　run through the day／終日行われている　mindfulness／心を込め，集中して物事を行える状態　metabolic rate／代謝率　a state of maximum efficiency／効率性が最大となる状態　after all／なにしろ〜だから　cope with 〜／〜にうまく対処する　food shortage／食料不足　be in safe hands／しっかり管理されて　On arrival at 〜／〜に到着するとすぐに　a consultation with a doctor／医師の診察　blood pressure／血圧　crisis day／一番苦しく大変な日　withdrawn／自分の中に閉じこもったような　light-headed／頭のくらくらする，朦朧とした　revelation／悟りを開いたような気持ち　clear-eyed／目の澄んだ　break the fast／断食を解く　tiny amounts of solid food／ごく少量の固形食　"good" cholesterol／善玉コレステロール　in the right ratio／適切な割合で　cortisol／コルチゾール（ストレスに反応して分泌されるホルモン）　joint pain／関節の痛み　calorie restriction／カロリー制限　adjustment／調整　The idea is that 〜／要は（大事なのは）〜だ

your body will undergo profound changes that last after the fast is ended. Improvements can be maintained through diet and by making fasting a normal part of life – as it once was.

Most impressive among the people I talked to at the clinic were the regular visitors for rheumatism and arthritis. Quite a number are fortunate enough to have the resources to come a couple of times a year, to fast for two weeks each time, and they have seen a drastic reduction in medication and pain, and a significant increase in joint mobility. The answer seems to lie with fasting's ability to decrease intestinal permeability – the "leaky gut" problem so often associated with inflammatory diseases, as large molecules acting as antigens pass through the intestinal wall and cause immune reactions. Eighty per cent of our immune system is in our gut. If the gut is wrong, we are wrong. Fasting is good for your gut.

I would like to experience the profound sense of wellbeing and peace of mind that fasting delivered again. And I had more time – think how much time shopping, cooking, eating and clearing up afterwards takes out of every day. Suddenly there was time to think deeply, to read, reassess, be with yourself, and to make a new friend of your body.

Notes:

profound change／重大な変化　impressive／印象に残っている　arthritis／関節炎　quite a number (of people)／かなり多数(の人)　resources／(通例，複数形で)資産，資金　a drastic reduction in ～／～の大幅な減少　medication／投薬　a significant increase in ～／～の著しい向上　joint mobility／関節の可動性　lie with ～／～にある　intestinal permeability／腸の透過性　the "leaky gut" problem／あのいわゆる「漏れやすい腸」の問題(＝Leaky Gut Syndrome (LGS),腸管壁浸漏症候群)　associated with ～／～の原因の１つとされる　inflammatory disease／炎症性疾患　molecule／分子　antigen／抗原　intestinal wall／腸壁　immune reaction／免疫反応　profound sense of wellbeing／心の底からの深い幸福感　peace of mind／心の安らぎ　clearing up／(食事の)後片付け　reassess／自分を見直す　be with yourself／自分とつき合う

練習問題

A 次の英文が，本文の内容と一致する場合にはT，一致しない場合にはFを（　）内に記入しなさい。

1. （　）While fasting, the body burns something unneeded along with healthy cells to generate heat and energy.
2. （　）Diseases linked to the immune system like asthma can be effectively treated through fasting.
3. （　）You should take exercise during the fast to raise the metabolic rate and keep it high.
4. （　）You can eat as much as you like soon after you break the fast.
5. （　）The body will go through radical changes while fasting, but the good effects will soon disappear after the fast is over.

B 音声を聴いて，次の英文の（　）内に適語を記入しなさい。　track 35～39

1. A charitable foundation for children with cancer (　　　)(　　　)(　　　) in 2010.
2. The old couple (　　　)(　　　) a small pension.
3. The final decision (　　　)(　　　) his parents.
4. Our (　　　)(　　　) is to help people in need.
5. If that is really what you want, you should (　　　)(　　　) it.

C 和文に合うように，（　）内の語句を並べかえて英文をつくりなさい。

1. 彼はお金のためなら何でもするような人間だ。
   (someone, money, would, is, kill, he, for, who).

2. かなり多くの人がそのビルの建設に反対している。
   (of, oppose, the building, a, people, quite, of, the construction, number).

3. われわれの会社は設備コストを大幅に削減する必要がある。
   (cost, needs, our, drastic, in, company, a, facility, reduction).

4. ストレスの多い状況に対処する方法についてのワークショップが，明日開催される。
   (tomorrow, a workshop, situations, there, cope, is, on, with, to, stressful, how).

5. その国では，高タンパク，高脂肪の食事に関連した病気にかかっている人が多い。
   (high-protein, high-fat, the country, a, many, associated, diet, people, health problems, with, have, and, in).

D 次の英語に相当する日本語を下から選び，記号で答えなさい。

1. septicaemia （ ） 2. gerontology （ ）
3. metabolic rate （ ） 4. arthritis （ ）
5. antigen （ ） 6. inflammatory disease （ ）
7. chronic rheumatism （ ） 8. immune system （ ）
9. pharmaceutical (*n.*) （ ） 10. toxin （ ）

a. 毒素	b. 慢性リウマチ	c. 炎症性疾患
d. 老年学	e. 敗血症	f. 関節炎
g. 製薬会社	h. 抗原	i. 免疫系
j. 代謝率		

Unit 6　37

Unit 7
偏った食習慣が病気を招く:味覚障害からうつ病まで

Low Zinc Levels Tied to Dulled Sense of Taste: Unbalanced Eating Habits May Cause Zinc Deficiency

The Japan News, April 11, 2015

track 40

Last October, a 46-year-old instructor at a confectionery school in Tokyo wondered why she couldn't taste the sweetness in a cake one of her students had made. The student had used the right ingredients. Around the same time, her husband began saying the taste of her miso soup and simmered dishes was too strong. She started meticulously following her recipe books and using measuring spoons. "If I can't taste things properly, I can't keep my job," she thought.

In early December, she went to see a doctor at Kashiwa Clinic in Kashiwa, Chiba Prefecture, after reading about a taste disorder on the clinic's website. At the clinic, sweet, salty, sour and bitter samples were placed on her tongue to see what concentrations of the sensations she could react to. She also had a blood test done to check her concentrations of zinc.

Tastes are perceived by taste buds and cells in the tongue and throat, and transmitted to the brain through nerves. Many strange and unfamiliar tastes are caused by a decline in the functioning of these taste buds in their capacity as sensors. Zinc is related to the metabolic system of taste buds, and a zinc deficiency can lead to a dulling of the sense of taste.

In the case of the confectionery school instructor, the zinc concentration in her blood

Notes:

zinc／亜鉛　sense of taste／味覚　unbalanced eating habits／バランスの悪い食習慣　deficiency／欠乏, 不足　instructor／講師　confectionery school／製菓専門学校　ingredient／（料理の）材料　around the same time／同じ頃　miso soup／味噌汁　simmered dishes／煮物　meticulously／細心の注意を払って　recipe book／料理本　measuring spoon／計量スプーン　properly／正しく　keep one's job／仕事を続ける　taste disorder／味覚障害　place／置く　tongue／舌　concentration／濃度　sensation／知覚（この場合, 味覚）　react to ～／～に反応する　blood test／血液検査　have A done／A（物）を～してもらう　perceive／知覚する　taste bud／味蕾（みらい）　cell／細胞　throat／喉　transmit／伝える　nerve／神経　decline／衰え, 低下　functioning／機能　capacity／能力　sensor／感知器（センサー）　be related to ～／～と関係している　metabolic system／代謝系　lead to ～／～をもたらす　dulling／鈍化

was on the lower end of the normal range, and she also had a shortage of iron. Unable to find any other cause, she began to undergo treatment to increase her zinc levels. A balance must be achieved between zinc and iron. When zinc is supplemented, iron levels decrease even further, which leads to a higher risk of anemia. After taking an iron supplement for about one month, she began to take medication containing zinc.

After about a month of taking zinc, her sense of taste gradually returned and she also became able to trust her tongue as she had before regarding seasonings. Test findings on her blood and tongue returned to normal.

Zinc is contained in many foods, such as meat or eggs. As long as you don't have an unbalanced diet or rely too much on instant or processed foods, you should have no problems with a deficiency.

The confectionery instructor had been extremely busy around the time she noticed her sense of taste was out of whack. She would have cake from her workplace for lunch, and for dinner she often made do with ready-made soups. Looking back, she said, "It might have been my horrible eating habits that left me zinc-deficient."

A taste disorder test takes about 30 minutes. The test yields little or no revenue for medical institutions, so only a limited number conduct it. Even Kashiwa Clinic only accepts a maximum of three patients a week by reservation for taste disorder tests, to prevent them from interfering with treating regular patients.

If you feel you are losing your sense of taste, "you should first go to the nearest clinic to see if there's insufficient zinc or iron in your blood," said Yoko Muraoka, an otolaryngologist who is deputy director of the clinic. "You might have an illness that can affect your sense of taste, such as diabetes or a liver disease."

(個人名・民間団体名は改変しています)

Notes:

the lower end of the normal range／正常域の下限　shortage of iron／鉄分不足　(be) unable to ～／～することができない　undergo／(治療などを)受ける　treatment／治療　supplement／補う　even further／さらにもっと　anemia／貧血　iron supplement／鉄分補給剤　medication／薬剤　gradually／次第に　trust／信用する　regarding ～／～に関して　seasoning／調味料　findings／調査結果　contain／含む　such as ～／～のような　as long as ～／～する限りは　rely on ～／～に頼る　processed food／加工食品　extremely／極めて　out of whack／調子が狂って　would ／よく～した(過去の短期的な習慣・反復行動)　workplace／仕事場　make do with ～／～で済ます，間に合わせる　ready-made／でき合いの　It might have been ～ that ...／…したのは，～だったかもしれない　yield／(利益などを)生み出す　little or no ～／ほとんど～ない　revenue／収益　medical institution／医療施設　conduct／おこなう　maximum／最大限　by reservation for ～／～を予約して　prevent A from ～ ing／Aが～しないようにする　interfere with ～／～を防げる　insufficient／不十分な　otolaryngologist／耳鼻咽喉科医　deputy director／副院長　diabetes／糖尿病　liver disease／肝臓病

Unbalanced Eating Habits, a Cause of Depression

The Japan News, May 30, 2015

track 41

Many people with depression are, in fact, suffering from metabolic syndrome. Recent studies have shown that psychological conditions such as depression are sometimes caused by unbalanced eating habits that lead to obesity or lack of nutrition. To combat this, hospitals have been increasing efforts to educate patients on food and nutrition. I visited the National Center of Neurology and Psychiatry in Kodaira, Tokyo, to find out more about the wide range of their projects, from research into the basics of nutrition to nutrition education for outpatients.

The center has a nutritional management office, which has seen an increase in the number of patients seeking nutrition education classes on scheduled psychiatric outpatient clinic days. Recently, many patients are seen showing photos saved on their smartphones of all the meals they had prior to the visit to the office's manager, Hiroshi Imai, or other nutritionists.

"What do you think? I tried really hard," said one patient, to which a nutritionist responded: "Looks great. You had plenty of vegetables." When patients have had three proper meals a day, with relatively small portions of rice and plenty of fruit and vegetables, Imai praises them. Patients are not asked to count calories because the task is deemed onerous.

"Even when you have a bento from a convenient store, you can easily add a side dish of vegetables, or have some vegetable juice without added sugar, to improve the nutritional balance of your meal," Imai said. "Many of our patients live alone so it is important for them to be able to work on their diet continually and with ease." People who suffer from depression typically have an unstable lifestyle, especially when it

Notes:

depression／うつ（症状）　in fact／実際には　suffer from ～／～に苦しむ　metabolic syndrome／メタボリックシンドローム（代謝症候群）　recent studies／最近の研究　psychological／心理的な　A such as B／BのようなA　obesity／肥満　lack of nutrition／栄養不足　the National Center of Neurology and Psychiatry／国立精神・神経医療研究センター　find out／解明する　the wide range of ～／広範囲の～　outpatient／外来患者　nutritional management office／栄養管理部　psychiatric outpatient clinic days／精神科外来日　prior to ～／～より前に　nutritionist／栄養士　plenty of ～／たくさんの～　relatively small portions of ～／比較的少量の～　calorie／カロリー　deem ～ onerous／～を面倒だと考える　convenient store／コンビニ　side dish／副菜　work on ～／～に取り組む　with ease／簡単に　unstable lifestyle／不安定な生活習慣

concerns meals.

In one case, an overweight man suffering from depression who habitually had extra meals late at night had difficulty getting up in the morning. Imai instructed him to have early evening meals and also to go to sleep earlier. This change gradually helped the man lose weight, become more active, and recover from depression.

People tend to have the impression that patients suffering from depression cannot eat well and lose weight because of that. Actually, many patients tend to be overweight with high neutral fat and blood sugar levels, according to research done by the center's Mental Disorder Research Department Director Hiroki Kume and others. A part of the brain that regulates our desire for food and drink also controls our stress levels. This explains why patients could be overweight due to stress.

It has also been pointed out that metabolic disorders, such as diabetes, can cause a minor but chronic inflammation of tissue, thereby increasing the risk of developing depression or lowering the function of insulin, which is known to reduce blood sugar levels. The latter can have a detrimental effect on brain function.

Nutrition deficiency can have other psychological effects. For example, it has been learned that iron deficiency can cause a variety of symptoms including poor concentration, fatigue and irritation. Postnatal depression, which can be experienced after giving birth and losing a large amount of blood, has been correlated to iron deficiency. "Although it is not always effective for everyone suffering from postnatal depression, many people do recover after taking iron supplements," Kume said.

There are many nutrients that are related to psychological conditions. For instance, a deficiency in folic acid, which is found in great quantities in green and yellow vegetables and influences the function of neurotransmitters, can lead to loss of motivation. But it is

Notes:

concern／(～に)関係している　overweight／太りすぎの　habitually／習慣的に　have difficulty getting up／起きるのが難しい　instruct A to ～／A（人）に～するよう教える　lose weight／減量する　tend to ～／～する傾向がある　because of ～／～が原因で　neutral fat／中和脂肪　blood sugar level／血糖値　according to ～／～によると　Mental Disorder Research Department Director／精神疾患研究センター長　regulate／統制する　due to ～／～が原因で　point out／指摘する　metabolic disorder／代謝障害　diabetes／糖尿病　chronic／慢性の　inflammation of tissue／組織の炎症　thereby／その結果　insulin／インスリン　the latter／後者　detrimental／有害な　iron deficiency／鉄分不足　a variety of ～／さまざまな～　symptom／症状　poor concentration／集中力低下　fatigue／疲労　irritation／イライラ　postnatal depression／産後うつ　give birth／出産する　a large amount of ～／多量の～　be correlated to ～／～と関連付けられる　iron supplement／鉄補充剤　nutrient／栄養素　folic acid／葉酸　in great quantities／多量に　neurotransmitter／神経伝達物質　loss of motivation／ヤル気の喪失

necessary to be aware that there are also some nutrients that can cause harm to the body when taken in excess through supplements.

Medical treatment for depression has typically comprised two aspects: drug therapy and counseling. But Kume said, "Like lifestyle-related diseases, it's also important that we carefully provide instruction on food, nutrition, and exercise for patients with depression."

（個人名・民間団体名は改変しています）

Notes:

be aware that 〜／〜ということに気づく　in excess／過剰に　medical treatment／治療　comprise／（〜から）成る
aspect／局面　drug therapy and counseling／薬物治療とカウンセリング　lifestyle-related disease／生活習慣病
instruction／指示　exercise／運動

練習問題

A 次の英文が，本文の内容と一致する場合にはT，一致しない場合にはFを（　）内に記入しなさい。

1. （　）There is an association between blood zinc levels and the sense of taste.
2. （　）Because a taste disorder test takes time, many hospitals are unwilling to conduct it.
3. （　）If you cannot identify tastes, there is a possibility that you develop diabetes.
4. （　）Food and nutrition education is necessary for patients with depression because unbalanced eating habits sometimes cause the condition.
5. （　）Patients suffering from depression tend to be overweight due to iron deficiency.

B 音声を聴いて，次の英文の（　）内に適語を記入しなさい。　track 42〜46

1. Internet addiction （　　）（　　）（　　） attention deficit in high school students.
2. The first step is （　　）（　　）（　　） the patient has a shortage of iron.
3. The drug has （　　）（　　）（　　） effect on cancer treatment.
4. The treatment （　　）（　　）（　　）（　　） for every patient.
5. Some nutrients can cause harm to the body （　　）（　　）（　　）（　　）.

C 和文に合うように，（　）内の語句を並べかえて英文をつくりなさい。

1. 関連のサイトにアクセスできなかったので，宿題するのをあきらめた。
   (gave up, access, I, unable, homework, a related-website, to, doing).

2. 彼の皮膚症状を悪化させたのは，不健康な食習慣だったかもしれない。
   (his unhealthy eating habits, been, the skin condition, it, have, worsened, might, that).

3. 子どもたちが加工食品に依存しすぎないようにしなければならない。
   (relying, prevent, processed foods, from, should, on, we, too much, children).

4. 彼は果物や野菜がたくさん入った食事を1日3回取るべきだといわれた。
   (three meals, fruit and vegetables, have, plenty of, he, to, a day, told, with, was).

5. 弟は朝早く起きるのが苦手だった。
   (had, early, my brother, getting up, in the morning, difficulty).

D 次の英語に相当する日本語を下から選び，記号で答えなさい。

1. ingredient	( )	2. deficiency	( )
3. seasoning	( )	4. concentration	( )
5. medication	( )	6. psychological	( )
7. nutrition	( )	8. psychiatric	( )
9. chronic	( )	10. symptom	( )

   a. 薬物   b. 精神科の   c. 欠乏
   d. 栄養   e. 症状   f. 心理的な
   g. 慢性の   h. 調味料   i. 成分
   j. 濃度

Unit 8
エボラ出血熱生存者たちの苦しみ

Many Ebola Survivors Struggling with Ailments
Voice of America, August 23, 2015　　Associated Press

 track 47

DAKAR, SENEGAL—

Lingering health problems afflicting many of the roughly 13,000 Ebola survivors have galvanized global and local health officials to find out how widespread the ailments are, and how to remedy them.

The World Health Organization calls it an emergency within an emergency.

Many of the survivors have vision and hearing issues. Some others experience physical and emotional pains, fatigue and other problems.

The medical community is negotiating uncharted waters as it tries to measure the scale of this problem that comes on the tail end of the biggest Ebola outbreak in history.

Future help

"If we can find out this kind of information, hopefully we can help other Ebola survivors in the future," Dr. Zan Yeong, an eye specialist involved in a study of health problems in survivors in Liberia, told The Associated Press.

About 7,500 people will enroll—1,500 Ebola survivors and 6,000 of their close contacts—and will be monitored over a five-year period in the study launched by Partnership for Research on Ebola Vaccines in Liberia, or PREVAIL.

Notes:

Ebola (disease) ／エボラ(出血熱)　survivor／生存者，回復者　struggle with ～／～と奮闘する　ailment／病気，不快　Associated Press／AP通信社 (1848年に設立された，アメリカに本拠を置く世界最古で最大の通信社)　lingering／長引く，なかなか消えない　afflict／(精神的／肉体的に)悩ませる，苦しめる　galvanize／衝撃を与える　health official／保健担当官　find out／探りだす，情報を得る　widespread／広範囲に及ぶ　remedy／治療する　the World Health Organization／世界保健機関(WHO)　emergency／緊急事態　issue／(個人的な)問題　physical／肉体的な　emotional／感情的な，情緒的な　fatigue／疲労，倦怠感　the medical community／医学界　negotiate／処理する，取り組む　uncharted waters／未知の領域 (unchartedは元来「海図に載っていない」を意味する)　measure／測定する，評価する　scale／規模，程度　the tail end／最終段階　outbreak／(疫病などの)大流行，急激な発生　hopefully／願わくば　in the future／将来は　involved in ～／～に関係する　health problem／健康問題　enroll／登録する　close contact／密接な接触(者)　over a five-year period／5年間にわたる　launch／(事業などを)開始する　Partnership for Research on Ebola Vaccines in Liberia／リベリア(共和国)におけるエボラ・ワクチンに関するパートナーシップ研究

Only about 40 percent of those infected have survived Ebola, according to WHO estimates. But while the survivors beat the odds, preliminary research shows that many are still suffering.

Around half those who received post-recovery check-ups have joint pain, said Dr. Daniel Bausch, an Ebola expert and consultant for WHO.

"We don't have the capacity yet—we wish we did—to follow every survivor," he said. Consequently, the percentage of survivors who have complications isn't known, Bausch said.

He described the joint pain as "very debilitating and a very serious problem that can prevent people from going back to work and providing for their family."

Quarter of survivors

Some degree of changes in vision has been reported by roughly 25 percent of the survivors who have been seen by medics, he said, including severe inflammation of the eye that if untreated can result in blindness, he said.

The Ebola virus has been found, in at least a few cases, to linger in the eyes, though experts say it is not transmitted through tears.

Morris Kallon, 34, a health worker who survived Ebola in a village in Liberia's Grand Cape Mount County, said he had fevers, headaches, lower abdominal pain and red eyes after he returned home.

"I have been experiencing a whole lot of problems within my body system," he said. "I still feel pains in my back. It is very difficult for me to swing my arms. ... My vision is always blurred, like dew on my face."

Lab technician Mohamed SK Sesay was working at a hospital in Kenema, a town in eastern Sierra Leone, testing blood samples for Ebola when he fell sick with the virus.

About eight members of his team got infected and he was among the few survivors, WHO said.

After he recovered, Sesay was discharged from an Ebola treatment unit in September. He was still weak, and says he was shunned by his community. Then his health deteriorated.

"Sleepless nights. Joint pain. Muscle pain," Sesay said. "I started experiencing loss of weight. ... Loss of sight was the worst one that set me off. I used to cry. I couldn't see my computer."

Eye health

He was attended to by one of Sierra Leone's few eye doctors and his health improved overall, but he still has bad days.

"My biggest challenge is now my health," Sesay said. He loses vision from time to time. Sometimes if people call out to him on the street, he can't hear them.

Eye problems were noted in some survivors of Ebola outbreaks in Congo in 1995, in Uganda's Gulu district in 2000 and in Uganda's Bundibugyo district in 2007. But with such small numbers, past outbreaks haven't provided sufficient opportunities for extensive study, Bausch said.

Now, with thousands of survivors, doctors want to learn why people are experiencing these ailments, how they affect the body, what percentage of survivors has issues and how to treat them.

Experts also want to learn whether the physical problems are directly caused by the virus, whether they existed before, are side-effects or perhaps autoimmune reactions, Bausch said.

"It's too early ... to know what the direct effect or link is to Ebola, if at all," Bausch said.

Notes:

he was among the few survivors／数少ない生存者のうちのひとりだった　recover／（健康を）回復する　be discharged from ～／～から退院する　Ebola treatment unit／エボラ(出血熱)治療施設　shun／疎外する　deteriorate／悪化する　loss of weight／体重減少　set A off／Aを怒らせる　used to ～／以前は～したものだ　be attended to／治療を受ける　overall／全体としては　challenge／試練　from time to time／時々　call out to ～／大声で～によびかける　on the street／路上で　Congo／コンゴ地域(中央アフリカの地域で，現在はコンゴ共和国，コンゴ民主共和国，カビンダの3カ国がある)　Uganda／ウガンダ共和国　extensive／大規模な，広範囲にわたる　thousands of ～／何千もの～　affect／(病気などが)冒す　whether／(～する)かどうか　side-effects／副作用　autoimmune reaction／自己免疫反応　if at all／仮にあったとしても

In early August, WHO gathered experts in Sierra Leone who concluded that more needs to be done to provide better care plans for survivors, and more research and specialist help is needed.

Post-recovery problems haven't been confined to West African survivors, whose health might not have been strong to begin with considering the poor state of health care in Liberia, Sierra Leone and Guinea—the three impoverished countries most affected by Ebola—even before the epidemic.

American survivors

Dr. Ian Crozier, an American who became infected while working in Sierra Leone for WHO, developed an inflammation and very high blood pressure in one eye months after being released from treatment.

His iris temporarily changed color from blue to green; doctors found his eye contained the Ebola virus. He is still recovering, but his vision has improved, according to Emory University Hospital which has been treating him.

Nancy Writebol, who last year became the second American infected with Ebola, said she suffers joint pain, mostly in her knees. She said she had problems with her vision, but they seem to have gone away.

Writebol assists a weekly survivor clinic in Liberia at ELWA hospital run by Serving In Mission, a North Carolina-based Christian organization.

She noted that Liberia's health care system is broken and many survivors lack running water and electricity in their homes, making their recovery more arduous than that of survivors in the West.

"There are a lot that are having troubles with vision," she said. "One of the greatest complaints that we see is joint pain. And you can tell just by the way people are moving that they are suffering."

Notes:

conclude／結論を下す　more needs to be done／さらに必要なことを行わなければならない　care plan／（医療）ケア計画　be confined to ~／~に限定される　to begin with／まず第一に　considering ~／~を考えると，~のわりには　poor state of ~／~の貧弱な状況　health care／健康管理　Guinea／ギニア共和国　impoverished／貧しい　epidemic／（病気などの）流行　high blood pressure／高血圧　release／解放する　iris／（眼球の）光彩　Emory University Hospital／エモリー大学病院（アメリカジョージア（Georgia）州アトランタ市（Atlanta）に所在する）　knee／ひざ　Serving In Mission／サービング・イン・ミッション（略してSIMともよばれる，アメリカに本部があり，国際的に活動するキリスト宣教団体）　North Carolina-based／ノース・カロライナ州に本拠を置く　running water／水道水　arduous／困難な，努力を要する　the West／西洋，欧米　complaint／不満の種　you can tell just by the way people are moving／人々の歩き方だけでわかる

Dr. Rick Sacra, an American Ebola survivor who helps at the ELWA Liberia hospital every few months, said when he was in Liberia in June and July, he saw a mixture of depression and post-traumatic stress disorder in the 15 to 40 people that came to survivor clinic appointments each week.

Physically, the main complaints involve the eyes, joints and nerve problems, Sacra said. Less common symptoms are rashes, headaches, abdominal discomfort and cough.

Some complications

"I know there's likely a large number of survivors who are fine, but then you have smaller subsets who have one or more of these complications," he said.

Sacra also suffered eye problems that were treated with steroids. He told AP he has fully recovered.

The epidemic, which has claimed nearly 11,300 lives, has significantly slowed, with only three confirmed cases emerging in the last weekly reporting period, according to WHO figures. But experts and survivors say the struggle to deal with the residual damage is just starting.

Dr. Anders Nordstrom, the WHO representative for Sierra Leone, said: "It is increasingly clear that emerging from an ETU (Ebola treatment unit) is just the beginning."

Notes:

every few months／2，3カ月ごとに　a mixture of ～／～の入り交じったもの　depression／うつ病，抑うつ症　post-traumatic stress disorder (PTSD) ／心的外傷後ストレス障害　nerve／神経　symptom／症状　rash／発疹　abdominal discomfort／腹部不快感　cough／咳　likely／たぶん～であろう　a large number of ～／多数の～　subset／小集団，一部（数学でいう「部分集合」をさす）　steroid／ステロイド薬（副腎皮質ホルモン中の「糖質コルチコイド」からつくられ，炎症やアレルギー反応を抑える治療薬として使われる）　AP（= Associated Press）／AP通信社　claim／（命を）奪う　significantly／著しく　confirmed／確認された　emerge／出る　WHO figure／WHOの関係者(figureには「～の人」の意味があり，a public figure（「著名人」）のように使われる）　deal with ～／～に取り組む　residual damage／まだ説明のつかない被害　representative／代表者

練習問題

A 次の英文が，本文の内容と一致する場合にはT，一致しない場合にはFを（　）内に記入しなさい。

1. (　) Around half of the Ebola survivors who received post-recovery check-ups have eye problems.
2. (　) Mohamed SK Sesay was among the few Ebola survivors at a hospital in Sierra Leone.
3. (　) Doctors want to learn why many Ebola survivors are experiencing the ailments.
4. (　) Post-recovery problems of Ebola have been confined to West African survivors.
5. (　) According to WHO, Ebola has significantly slowed.

B 音声を聴いて，次の英文の（　）内に適語を記入しなさい。　　track 48～52

1. Many people have to (　　　) (　　　) finding a good work-life balance.
2. I believe that you have the courage to venture into (　　　) (　　　).
3. The health care system of this country has (　　　) (　　　) (　　　) (　　　) problems.
4. (　　　) (　　　) people gathered to celebrate the end of the Ebola epidemic.
5. The recent hurricane (　　　) (　　　) a loss of just over 100 million dollars.

C 和文に合うように，（　）内の語句を並べかえて英文をつくりなさい。

1. 彼がいまどこにいるかみつけてもらえますか。
   (is, could, right now, he, out, where, you, find)?

2. 自分の夢を叶えるために，ヘンリーは逆境に打ち勝たねばなりません。
   (order, Henry, to, beat, his dream, has to, capture, the odds, in).

3. 私たちの懸命な努力はコンテストで1位という結果になりました。
　　(resulted, the first, excellent, of, in, the contest, our, effort, prize).

4. 彼女は2週間後に退院しました。
　　(discharged, hospital, the, she, from, weeks, was, two, after).

5. 世界はもっと積極的に地球温暖化に取り組まなければなりません。
　　(aggressively, warming, with, the world, global, must, deal, more).

D 次の略語が意味する英語表記を下の選択肢から選んで（　）内に記号で記入し、さらにその日本語の意味を［　］内に書きなさい。

	英語表記	日本語
1. BG	(　)	[　]
2. AIDS	(　)	[　]
3. HIV	(　)	[　]
4. TB	(　)	[　]
5. CT	(　)	[　]
6. DM	(　)	[　]
7. GU	(　)	[　]
8. QOL	(　)	[　]
9. ECG	(　)	[　]
10. PTSD	(　)	[　]

> a) electrocardiogram　　b) tuberculosis　　c) post-traumatic stress disorder
> d) computerized tomography　　e) human immunodeficiency virus
> f) diabetes mellitus　　g) blood glucose　　h) quality of life
> i) gastric ulcer　　j) acquired immunodeficiency syndrome

Unit 9

誰でもできる健康レシピ

Herbs and Spices May Improve Your Health
Voice of America, July 9, 2013

track 53

People have been using herbs and spices for thousands of years. Generally, herbs come from the green leaves of plants or vegetables. Spices come from other parts of plants and trees. Some herbs and spices are valued for their taste. They help to sharpen the taste of many foods. Others are chosen for their smell. Still others were used traditionally for health reasons.

When people think of improving their diet, they often talk about eating more fruits and vegetables. Others want to eat more fish and less red meat, in addition to reducing the amount of food they eat. But, they can improve their diets even more with just a simple addition.

Penn State Associate Professor Sheila West led an investigation of the health effects of a spice-rich diet. Her team knew that a high-fat meal produces high levels of triglycerides, a kind of fat, in the blood.

She said, "If this happens too frequently, or if triglyceride levels are raised too much, your risk of heart disease is increased. We found that adding spices to a high-fat meal reduced triglyceride response by about 30 percent, compared to a similar meal with no spices added."

As part of the study, her team prepared meals on two separate days for six men between the ages of 30 and 65. The men were overweight, but healthy. The researchers added about 30 milliliters of spices to each serving of the test meal, which included chicken curry, Italian herb bread and a cinnamon biscuit. The meal for the control group

Notes:

herb／薬草　spice／スパイス　thousands of ～／何千もの～　Some herbs ～ . Others ～ . Still others ～ . ／～な薬草もあれば～な薬草もある。さらに～な薬草もあった。　value／評価する　sharpen／鋭敏にする　think of ～／～について考える　diet／食事　red meat／赤身の肉　in addition to ～／～に加えて　amount／量　addition／追加　investigation／研究　spice-rich diet／スパイスを多く含んだ食事　high-fat meal／高脂肪分を含んだ食事　triglyceride／トリグリセリド（脂肪組織の主成分）　frequently／しばしば　risk／危険性　heart disease／心臓病　response／反応，感応　compared to ～／～と比較して　prepare／準備する　overweight／太りすぎの　researcher／研究者　cinnamon／シナモン（乾燥させ粉末にした黄褐色の桂皮）

was the same, but it did not include any spices.

Ann Skulas-Ray also served on the research team. She said the team used paprika, rosemary, oregano, cinnamon, turmeric, black pepper, cloves and garlic powder. She said these spices were chosen because they had demonstrated strong antioxidant activity under controlled conditions in a laboratory.

During the experiment, the researchers removed blood from the men every 30 minutes for three hours. They found that antioxidant activity in the blood of the men who ate the spicy meal was 13 percent higher than it was for the men who did not. In addition, insulin activity dropped by about 20 percent in the men who ate the spicy food.

Professor West says, "Antioxidants, like spices, may be important in reducing oxidative stress and thus reducing the risk of chronic disease." She adds that the level of spices used in the study provided the same amount of antioxidants found in 150 milliliters of red wine or about 38 grams of dark chocolate.

Pepper may help you lose weight

Other scientists are helping to uncover the secrets of spices and herbs. For example, Purdue University researchers in Indiana say red pepper may help people lose weight. They say this could be especially true for people who do not usually add peppers to their food.

The researchers reported on the effects of dried and ground cayenne red pepper in the journal *Physiology & Behavior* in 2011. They found that small changes in diet, like adding the pepper, may reduce the desire to eat.

Most chili peppers contain capsaicin -- a substance that makes chili peppers taste hot and spicy. Other studies have shown that capsaicin can reduce hunger and burn calories, the energy stored in food.

Notes:

include ～／～を含む　paprika／パプリカ(乾燥した赤色の粉末香辛料)　rosemary／ローズマリー(地中海原産のハッカ科の常緑低木の青みがかった葉で調味料，香料・医薬品として使う)　oregano／オレガノ(シソ科のハナハッカ属の多年草で葉に芳香があり，香味料として使う)　turmeric／ターメリック(カレーの材料)　clove／クローブ(チョウジの木の蕾を乾燥させたもので香料，生薬，肉料理によく用いる)　demonstrate／証明する　antioxidant activity／非酸化活動　laboratory／実験場　experiment／実験　remove A from B／BからAを取り除く　insulin activity／インシュリンの活動　oxidative／酸化の，酸化力のある　chronic disease／慢性疾患　provide ～／～に供給する，～に支給する　dark chocolate／ブラックチョコレート(ミルクがほとんど入っていない)　uncover ～／～を明らかにする　effect／効果　ground／粉末の　cayenne／カエニン(赤唐辛子の一種)　capsaicin／カプサイシン(唐辛子の成分)　substance／物質

Twenty-five people of normal weight took part in the study, which lasted six weeks. Thirteen of them liked spicy food. The 12 others did not. The researchers decided how much red pepper each group would receive. One and eight tenths grams of the pepper was given to each person who liked spicy food. The others received three tenths of a gram.

　The people who did not normally eat red pepper showed a decreased desire for food. That was especially true for fatty, salty and sweet foods. Purdue University Professor Richard Mattes said the effect may be true only for people who do not usually eat red pepper. He said the effectiveness of the pepper may be lost if spices are normally part of a person's diet and that more studies must be done.

　Other research shows that capsaicin helps suppress the buildup of body fat. A study published in the *American Journal of Clinical Nutrition* found that capsaicin may help to reduce abdominal fat. Study organizers said the reduction possibly takes place because the spice changes some proteins found in fat, causing them to break down the fat.

Spices may help fight disease

　Scientists have become so interested in the health value of spices that recent discoveries are helping to move spices from traditional medicine into real science.

　Researchers in Virginia discovered that curcumin, a substance found in turmeric, stopped the Rift Valley Fever virus from reproducing in infected cells. The sometimes deadly virus is carried by mosquitos. It can affect human beings and some farm animals like cattle and goats.

　A study published in the *Journal of Biological Chemistry* found that curcumin improves the effectiveness of chemotherapy in breast cancer patients. And it has possibilities for development into a drug that can help with chemotherapy.

　Turmeric comes from a tropical plant common to India. Scientists have been examining its medical possibilities for many years. Studies show that turmeric's qualities may help protect against damage to the body's tissues and other injuries. Researchers also said turmeric may reduce evidence of damage in the brains of patients with mild or

Notes:

take part in ～／～に参加する　last／続く　effectiveness／効果　suppress／抑制する　abdominal fat／お腹の周りの脂肪　reduction／減少　take place／起こる　protein／タンパク質　break down ～／～を壊す　so ～ that...／（結果を表して）非常に～なので…　curcumin／カレーの材料　Rift Valley Fever／リフト谷熱(蚊などが媒体する感染性の強いウイルス性疾患)　infected cell／感染した細胞　deadly virus／死にいたるウイルス　affect／影響する　chemotherapy／化学療法　breast cancer／乳がん　body's tissue／体の細胞組織

moderate Alzheimer's disease. For this reason, the researchers designed a study that examined results from a mental-performance test of older Asian adults.

The study involved curry, which contains turmeric. The adults tested were 60 to 93 years old. Those who sometimes ate curry did better on the tests than individuals who rarely or never ate curry. This was also true of those who ate it often or very often.

One spice that often is at the top of a healthy spices list is cinnamon. It comes from the inner bark of several trees and is used in both sweet and savory cooking. For centuries, cinnamon has been used in traditional medicine. Now, it is earning respect in the medical field.

German researchers found that cinnamon can reduce blood sugar by ten percent. They were not sure why, but said it could be that substances in cinnamon activate enzymes that excite insulin receptors. Research also shows the spice can help lower levels of cholesterol and triglycerides, blood fats that may cause diabetes.

Registered dietician Wendy Bazilian says spices are being considered more seriously because the added taste they bring helps people reduce the salt, fat and sugar in their cooking. She has written a book called, "The Super Foods Rx Diet", on how people can lose weight by basing their diet on what she calls "super nutrients". She says she likes oregano, for example, because she considers it a mini salad. She says "one teaspoon has as much antioxidant power as three cups of chopped broccoli." But, she says do not get rid of the broccoli. Instead, eat both.

Herbs and spices are not used just to lessen unwanted chemical effects. They make food taste better. Some spices also destroy bacteria. Spices have long been used to keep food safe to eat. Spices have influenced world history.

Notes:

Alzheimer's disease／アルツハイマー病　those who ～／～な人々　be true of ～／～に当てはまる　bark／木の皮　savory／食欲をそそる　blood sugar／血糖値　enzyme／酵素　excite／促進させる　insulin receptor／インスリン受容体　diabetes／糖尿病　registered dietician／管理栄養士　consider ～／～と考える　"super nutrients"／「最高の栄養」　chopped／細切れの　get rid of ～／～を取り除く　lessen／少なくする(lessの動詞形)　unwanted／必要のない　chemical effect／化学的な効果

練習問題

A 次の語句のうち，herb には（h）を，spice には（s）を，herb と spice の両方に用いられるものには（h/s）を書き入れなさい。

1. mint　　　　　　（　　）
2. cinnamon　　　（　　）
3. oregano　　　　（　　）
4. clove　　　　　（　　）
5. thyme　　　　　（　　）
6. ginger　　　　　（　　）
7. sansho　　　　　（　　）
8. paprika　　　　（　　）
9. garlic　　　　　（　　）
10. rosemary　　　（　　）
11. nutmeg　　　　（　　）
12. basil　　　　　（　　）
13. black pepper　（　　）
14. coriander　　　（　　）
15. turmeric　　　（　　）

B 音声を聴いて，次の英文の（　）内に適語を記入しなさい。　track 54～58

1. Herbs are the fresh and dried (　　　　) generally of temperate plants and are usually (　　　) in color.
2. Spices are the (　　　), fruit, seeds, bark, and roots typically of (　　　　) plants and range from brown to black to red in color.
3. Many scientists are helping to discover the (　　　　) of spices and herbs.
4. A group of scientists found that curcumin (　　　　) the effectiveness of chemotherapy in (　　　)(　　　) patients.
5. The cinnamon comes from the inner (　　　) of several trees and is used in both sweet and (　　　) cooking.

C 和文に合うように，（　）内の語句を並べかえて英文をつくりなさい。

1. 立派な人になりたいのなら，悪い習慣はすぐに止めるべきです。
   You should (to become, get, bad habits, if, a, immediately, your, refined, rid of, you, person, want).

2. これから取り付けたカテーテルを外します。
   (from, remove, I'm, your, equipment, going to, the, catheter).

3. ナンシーは自分の娘に，たくさんのお金を衣服につぎ込むことをやめさせようとした。
Nancy (spending, clothing, her, tried, a lot of, to stop, daughter, money, on, from).

4. 例年の音楽会は今月末に産業会館で行われる。
An annual (at, will, music concert, at the end, a convention center, of this month, take place).

5. 今日，スパイスは主に調味料目的で使用される乾燥した植物の製品として知られるようになった。
Today (primarily, known, spices, as, plant product, have become, seasoning purposes, for, any dried, used).

D 次の英語に相当する語句を下から選び，記号で答えなさい。

1. savory　　　　(　) 　　2. enzyme　　　　(　)
3. antioxidant　　(　) 　　4. protein　　　　(　)
5. Alzheimer's　　(　) 　　6. calorie　　　　(　)
7. chemotherapy　(　) 　　8. chronic disease　(　)

> a) the treatment of disease, especially cancer, with the use of chemical substances
> b) a natural substance found in meat, eggs, fish, some vegetables, etc.
> c) having a pleasant taste or smell
> d) a disease lasting for a long time, difficult to cure easily
> e) a unit of measuring how much energy food will produce
> f) a substance such as Vitamin C or E that removes dangerous molecules
> g) a serious disease, especially affecting older people's brain, causing loss of memory, loss of ability to speak clearly, etc.
> h) a substance, produced by all living things, which helps chemical change happen or happen more quickly, without being changed itself

Unit 10
成長を続けるティーンエイジャーの脳

Understanding the Teen Brain Key for Better Parenting
Voice of America, January 30, 2015

 track 59

Neuroscientist Frances Jensen has been studying the human brain for almost all of her career. But even she wasn't ready for the challenge of two teenage sons. Her challenge: try to find out why smart and responsible teenagers also act impulsively and engage in high-risk behaviors.

So, she did what any scientist would do... she studied a decade's worth of brain research. Her findings dispel some myths and also provide a bit of help for parents, teachers and other adults trying to understand.

Teen brain - a work in progress

When they reach puberty, their bodies change and teens look like adults. The assumption is their brain also is like an adult brain.

Not true, Jensen said. "The brain is the last organ in the body to mature. It takes into mid-20s for it to complete." The chemistry and structure of the teenaged brain is only about 80% of its final form.

In her new book, *The Teenage Brain: A Neuroscientist's Survival Guide to Raising Adolescents and Young Adults*, Jensen outlines the strengths and weaknesses of the brain at this stage of development. She said the way their brain is wired makes teens better learners than adults.

"It's coming down from a high on learning that happens in childhood, something we call 'synaptic plasticity,' which means that the synapses, where your brain cells talk to

---

Notes:

parenting ／子育て　neuroscientist ／神経科学者　challenge ／課題　impulsively ／衝動的に　engage in ～／～に携わる　～ worth of... ／～を要する…, ～分の…　dispel ／一掃する　myth ／通説　a bit of ～／少しの～　in progress ／進行中の　puberty ／思春期　assumption ／仮定, 前提　organ ／器官　mature ／十分に発達する　complete ／完成する　chemistry ／化学的性質　Adolescents and Young Adults ／思春期の人および若い成人　outline ／概要を述べる　at this stage of ～／～の段階で　be wired ／接続している　synaptic plasticity ／シナプス可塑性(シナプスは脳と体の情報伝達を担っている神経細胞同士の接合部。シナプスがその性質を変化させる能力を可塑性という。シナプス可塑性は記憶や学習に重要な役割を果たしている)　synapse ／シナプス　cell ／細胞

each other, are how you learn," said Jensen. "So you build bigger synapses when you learn something."

"The proteins and the chemicals involved in building synapses for learning are at very, very high levels in the child, and a little bit less in adolescents and then come down to sort of adult levels, which is why a child can learn two, three languages flawlessly and a teenager is pretty good, not quite as good as a child, but better than an adult in terms of the rate at which they can learn and absorb information."

The paradox is that while teens have an enhanced ability to learn, the connections among different areas of the brain are still developing.

"Your brain cells send out processes so that your brain areas can talk to each other. This process requires signals to go through the brain. These processes need insulation," said Jensen.

"And the insulation we have is a fatty natural substance called 'myelin.' It takes two-and-a-half decades to finish the job. They are working from the back of your brain to the front. And what do you think the last place to connect up fully to have these processes completed for fast transmission is? It's the front of your brain. And what's in the front of your brain? It's the frontal lobes," she said.

The frontal lobes of the brain are responsible for insight, judgment, impulse control and empathy, things a teenager has a hard time putting together.

"So we have a very active brain, on one hand, able to learn, but it's being driven by a driver who doesn't really have full access to the brakes yet," she said.

IQ and bad habits

Jensen says that things like drugs and alcohol can have a much more serious impact on the teen brain than the adult brain.

"Your IQ can change up or down between 13 and 17 years old. We don't quite know what specifically can make an IQ go up or down, but one thing that we know does

---

Notes:

protein／タンパク質　chemical／化学物質　(be) involved in ～／～に関与する　sort of／いわば，多少　flawlessly／完璧に　in terms of ～／～の観点から　absorb／吸収する　paradox／逆説　enhanced／高められた　send out ～／～を送り出す　so that S can ～／Sが～できるように　require A to ～／Aに～をするよう要求する　insulation／絶縁体　fatty／脂肪質の　substance／物質　myelin／ミエリン（神経細胞の軸索を取り囲む絶縁性の脂質層）　It takes（時間）to ～／～するのに（時間）がかかる　have A 過去分詞／Aを～させる　transmission／伝達　frontal lobe／前頭葉　insight／洞察力　impulse／衝動　empathy／共感　have a hard time ～ ing／～するのが困難である　on one hand／一方では　access to ～／～を利用する方法　IQ／知能指数（= intelligence quotient）　have an impact on ～／～に影響を与える　specifically／具体的に

make IQs go down is certainly exposure to certain drugs, for instance chronic pot smoking; the more you smoke, the lower your IQ will be between that time window."

So while we tend to think that teenagers are so resilient, neuroscientist Jensen said they are and they aren't.

"There are certain things that can affect them long term," she explained. "The same amount of experiences like stress or alcohol or pot, an adult may sail through it -- for the same exposure -- but a teenager will bear a long-term problem based on that."

Boys, girls and multitasking

A recent study reveals a short-term problem for teens: multi-tasking. That sensory overload can hinder their ability to recall words. "In this study," Jensen reported, "the ones who were given all sorts of distractions as they were trying to learn a task, they still did worse than the kids that were given the same learning experience without distraction. So teenagers can think, 'Oh, I can learn and do that all at the same time.' No, it's still an issue for their brain. There is a limit."

There is also a gender difference in brain development. Jensen said the part of the brain that processes information expands during childhood and then begins to thin, peaking in girls at around 12 to 14 years old and in boys about two years later. She compares a 13, 14 or 15 year-old-girl and a 13, 14 or 15 year-old boy.

"Of course there are individual exceptions, but we can say in general, the girls are probably more planners, able to sort of navigate through a complex sort of scheduling and things, whereas planning isn't a boy's big strength at this point of their life."

Sleepy brain

And while sleep is important for learning and memory, teens -- both boys and girls -- often don't get enough. When they stay up late at night and wake up late in the morning, parents may think it's just because teens are lazy.

That is another myth, Jensen says. They are just being teens. "Their biological clocks

---

Notes:

exposure to ～／～の影響をまともに受けること　chronic／常習的な　pot／マリファナ　the 比較級～, the 比較級…／～すればするほど，ますます…である　time window／期間　tend to ～／～する傾向がある　resilient／回復力がある　long term／長期間（short term = 短期間）　sail through ～／～を楽々と通過する　bear／抱える　based on ～／～に基づいて　multitasking／一度に複数の仕事をこなすこと　sensory／知覚の　overload／過重負担　hinder／妨げる　distraction／注意をそらせるもの　gender／ジェンダー（社会的・文化的観点からみた性差）　in general／一般に　navigate through ～／～を乗り越えていく　～ sort of...／～なタイプの…　whereas／それに反して　stay up late at night／夜ふかしをする　biological clock／体内時計

are absolutely programmed to be 2 to 3 hours later for the sleep start time and wake time than adults." Adults get a surge of melatonin, the hormone produced by the brain that helps make you sleepy, around 8:30. It typically doesn't hit teens until closer to 11 p.m. "So they're not ready to go to sleep yet until midnight," Jensen pointed out. "Likewise they have to go through the whole 8 to 9 hours of sleep in order to have a healthy brain." Waking up at 6:00 in the morning to get ready for school is like an adult getting up at 3:00 a.m.

"It's probably not the optimal time for their brains to be put in a learning environment," she said.

Parents: be patient and vigilant

All the new information about the teen brain can help adults do a better job as teachers and parents.

"Stay connected and also be a little bit more patient," Jensen advises adults. "This is the first generation in which we've known very much about the unique aspects of the adolescent brain; the strengths and weaknesses. Also, it's during these teenage years that mental illnesses can first strike: bi-polar, depression or schizophrenia. We see these things coming at 18, 19, 20 or early 20s. That's another reason to stay connected and know how to look for the warning signs."

Jensen also encourages parents to share such information with their kids. "In teenage years, they're trying to learn who they are, to figure out their identity. They have a natural interest in anything about themselves that can be told, so when you start telling them about the biology of their maturation state, you're surprised how quite interested in it they are."

Notes:

a surge of 〜／〜の急激な増加　melatonin／メラトニン（脳の松果体から分泌されるホルモンで体内時計を調整する）
hormone／ホルモン　close to 〜／〜近くに　point out 〜／〜を指摘する　likewise／そのうえ　optimal／最適な
vigilant／絶えず気を配っている　stay 〜／〜の状態のままでいる　bi-polar／双極性（障害）　depression／うつ病
schizophrenia／統合失調症　look for 〜／〜を探す　warning sign／（病気などの）前兆　figure out 〜／〜を理解する
biology of 〜／〜の生態，仕組み　maturation／成熟

練習問題

A 次の英文が，本文の内容と一致する場合にはT，一致しない場合にはFを（ ）内に記入しなさい。

1. （ ） Teenagers cannot manage their emotions well due to the undeveloped frontal lobes.
2. （ ） Teenagers' IQ will have no negative effects as long as they have the same amount of alcohol or pot as adults.
3. （ ） Jensen has found out that girls tend to reach a peak of brain information processing about two years younger than boys.
4. （ ） According to Jensen, teenagers should get up and go to bed early in order to make the most of their biological clocks.
5. （ ） Teenagers today are the first generation with unique aspects of the brain and with mental illnesses such as schizophrenia.

B 音声を聴いて，次の英文の（ ）内に適語を記入しなさい。　　track 60〜64

1. （　　　）（　　　）, we see an epidemic of influenza in winter.
2. （　　　）（　　　）（　　　） salt will make the soup taste better.
3. I have no complaints （　　　）（　　　）（　　　） my salary.
4. The student at last （　　　）（　　　） the solution to the math problem.
5. Don't （　　　）（　　　）（　　　） at night, or you won't get up on time.

C 和文に合うように，（ ）内の語句を並べかえて英文をつくりなさい。

1. 彼はかかりつけの歯科医院で歯垢を除去してもらった。
   (dentist's, had, office, he, at, removed, his family's, plaque).

2. 彼女はその仮説に欠点があると指摘した。
   (pointed, she, flaw, that, out, a, had, the hypothesis).

3. 飲酒量が増えれば増えるほど，アルコール依存症になる危険性はますます高くなる。
   (the risk you have, an alcoholic, you, the higher, alcohol, for becoming, the more, drink).

4. 数人の社員が新しい医療機器の開発に関与した。
   (developing, a, employees, were, in, new, device, involved, several, medical).

5. 悪いところはないと確かめることができるように，私は毎年健康診断を受ける。
   (I, is, medical checkup, have, I can, annual, wrong, be sure, nothing, so that, an).

D 次の英語に相当する日本語を下から選び，記号で答えなさい。
1. hippocampus   (　)
2. frontal lobe   (　)
3. parietal lobe   (　)
4. temporal lobe   (　)
5. occipital lobe   (　)
6. cerebrum   (　)
7. cerebellum   (　)
8. pituitary gland (　)
9. cranium   (　)
10. spinal cord   (　)

a. 脊髄	b. 大脳	c. 頭頂葉
d. 海馬	e. 頭蓋	f. 後頭葉
g. 前頭葉	h. 下垂体	i. 側頭葉
j. 小脳		

Unit 11

血圧と食生活の関係

Dietary Changes Help Lower Blood Pressure
Voice of America, April 5, 2013

track 65

　Sunday, April 7, is World Health Day, and this year's theme is high blood pressure, also known as hypertension. The World Health Organization has recommended reducing salt or sodium intake to lower the risk of stroke, cardiovascular disease and kidney failure. But researchers say the benefits would be greater if dietary potassium intake was increased at the same time.

　The WHO says high blood pressure affects one billion people worldwide. It leads to many deaths or permanent disabilities. Hypertension is called the silent killer because there are few obvious symptoms.

　The good news is it's often preventable. There are many studies indicating that reducing salt or sodium intake can lower the risk of stroke and related illnesses.

　Professor Graham MacGregor and his colleagues have reviewed past studies on salt intake and conducted their own.

　"When you eat more salt, the salt's absorbed into the body and then you get thirsty. You drink more water. As you know, salt makes you thirsty. That increases the amount of fluid around the cells because salt is the main regulator of the volume of fluid both in the circulation and the fluid around the cells – the so-called extra cellular volume. Now when that reaches a certain point, a message goes to the kidney that, hey, the body's got more salt in it. And then you start excreting in the urine more salt. So you come back

Notes:

dietary／食事の　lower blood pressure／血圧を下げる　World Health Day／世界保健デー　theme／テーマ　high blood pressure／高血圧　hypertension／高血圧　the World Health Organization(WHO)／世界保健機関　sodium／ナトリウム　intake／摂取　stroke／(脳)卒中，発作　cardiovascular disease／心血管疾患　kidney failure／腎不全　dietary potassium／食事性カリウム　affect ～／～に悪影響を及ぼす　lead to ～／～につながる　permanent disability／恒久的な障害　silent killer／サイレント・キラー(あまり注目されないが，命取りになることが多い隠れた危険因子)　obvious／明白な　symptom／兆候　preventable／予防できる　study／研究　related illness／関連疾患　be absorbed into ～／～に吸収される　fluid／(体)液，液体　cell／細胞　regulator／調整装置　volume／量　circulation／循環　so-called／いわゆる　extra cellular volume／細胞外容量　a certain point／ある一定の点　kidney／腎臓　start excreting ～／～を排泄し始める　urine／尿　come back into balance／バランスの取れた状態に戻る

into balance," he said.

MacGregor is a professor of cardiovascular medicine at the Barts and London School of Medicine and Dentistry.

"When you're on the high salt intake you always have some extra salt in you and a slightly greater volume of blood. And that's what puts up the blood pressure. I mean, if you wanted, an analogous thing would be really like a central heating system. If you put more water into closed system, the pressure will go up."

The body does need some salt, he said, about less than half a gram per day. However, people in developed nations are eating about eight to ten grams a day.

"So we're eating about 20 times more salt than we need, but no mammal normally adds salt to their food. We're the only mammals that do. We've only been doing it about 5,000 years because it had this magic property of preserving food and was very important to the development of civilization. But without that discovery, we wouldn't be eating salt," he said.

Much of the processed food today contains high levels of salt. That in combination with high sugar content can make so-called junk food delicious, but not nutritious.

MacGregor said that lowering salt can go a long way to reducing hypertension, but he says there's more than can be done, namely, increasing potassium intake. Studies show that higher potassium intake has been linked with a 24 percent lower risk of strokes in adults and may have a beneficial effect on blood pressure in children.

"It's in fruit and vegetables and also in unprocessed meat and fish. Probably during evolution, we were eating two or three times the amount of potassium we eat [now]. And the food industry, of course, when it processes food, removes potassium and adds salt, which is the worst possible thing to do."

Potassium, he said, counteracts some of the effects of salt. It's also important for nerve function and muscle control. The general recommendation is to get it through food and not supplements. People in developed countries consume about three grams of

Notes:

cardiovascular medicine／循環器学　the Barts and London School of Medicine and Dentistry／バーツ・ロンドン医科歯科大学　be on ～／～（の状態で）いる　extra／余分な　put up ～／～を上げる　blood pressure／血圧　analogous／類似した　central heating system／集中暖房システム　closed system／閉鎖されたシステム　less than ～／～未満　developed nations／先進諸国　mammal／哺乳動物　property／特性　processed food／加工食品　in combination with ～／～との組み合わせにおける　high sugar content／高糖度　nutritious／栄養のある　go a long way to ～／～に大いに役に立つ　potassium intake／カリウム摂取　be linked with ～／～と繋がっている　beneficial effect／有益な作用　unprocessed／加工されていない　evolution／進化　counteract ～／～を中和する，～を妨害する　nerve function／神経機能　muscle control／筋肉制御　supplement／サプリメント　consume／消費する

potassium a day through diet.

"The recommendation is that we should eat about four grams. Now to increase your potassium by one gram is equivalent to two or three servings of fruits and vegetables. It's equivalent to two or three bananas or two or three oranges or an orange, an apple and a banana or a serving of a vegetable and two fruit servings," he said.

It sounds easy, but health officials say it can be difficult to get people to eat more fruits and vegetables. MacGregor says in Britain, despite spending millions of dollars on awareness campaigns, daily consumption of potassium has barely increased. But Britain has had some success in reducing dietary salt or sodium.

"Eighty percent of the salt we eat is courtesy of the food industry. We have no choice. It's already there. And what we've done in the U.K. is to get the food industry to slowly reduce the amount of salt they add to food. So salt intake in the U.K. has fallen from I think 9.5 grams a day to 8.1, which is about a 15 percent reduction, which will have saved I think 9,000 deaths a year from strokes and heart attacks," he said.

Professor MacGregor said that by gradually reducing salt in foods people are less likely to notice the taste difference.

Health officials are raising concerns about developing countries with growing economies. Those nations are adopting a western diet – with its salty, sugary and fatty foods. Officials are forecasting a sharp rise in cardiovascular disease, along with obesity-related illnesses.

Notes:

be equivalent to ～／～と同等である　serving／一人前　health official／保健担当官　spend A on B／AをBに費やす　millions of ～／数百万もの～　awareness campaign／啓蒙活動　consumption／消費（量）　barely／ほとんど～ない　courtesy／好意，優遇　heart attack／心臓発作　be less likely to ～／～する可能性が低い　growing economy／成長を続ける経済　fatty／脂っこい　sharp rise／急激な上昇　along with ～／～に加えて　obesity-related illness／肥満に関連した病気

Study: Packaged Food Contains Unhealthy Levels of Salt

Voice of America, April 3, 2015

track 66

A new study by the U.S. Centers for Disease Control and Prevention, or CDC, found that more than half of all packaged grocery items in the United States contain levels of salt in excess of government recommendations. The foods include those most commonly purchased by consumers.

Salt is a contributor to high blood pressure, which is a risk factor for heart disease.

Investigators with the CDC looked at the sodium or salt content in 10 packaged grocery items.

"We looked at bread, cold cuts, pizza, poultry, soup, sandwiches, cheese, pasta-mixed dishes, meat-mixed dishes and savory snacks," said Linda Scheib, an epidemiologist with the center's Division for Heart Disease and Stroke Prevention.

Scheib's team looked at the salt content of 3,800 food products that contribute the most sodium to the diet.

They found that up to 70 percent of cold cuts, soups and sandwiches have a salt content higher than the daily recommendation by the U.S. Food and Drug Administration.

Ten percent of snack food, breads and cheese exceed the FDA's recommended daily allowance.

Many foods that seem healthy, according to Scheib, are actually full of salt. She said "bread is the No. 1 contributor of sodium to diet."

"A lot of foods that people don't think taste salty do actually have a lot of sodium in them," she added. "So, we recommend people just read those nutrition labels, make

Notes:

the U.S. Centers for Disease Control and Prevention (CDC)／アメリカ疾病管理予防センター　packaged grocery items／包装食品　level of ～／～の水準　in excess of ～／～を超過して　contributor／貢献者　risk factor／危険因子　sodium content／ナトリウム含有量　salt content／塩分含有量　cold cuts／コールドカット（さまざまな種類のハム・ソーセージなどの冷肉の薄切り料理）　poultry／家禽（鶏・七面鳥・アヒル・ガチョウをさす）　pasta-mixed dishes／パスタ料理　meat-mixed dishes／肉料理　savory snacks／（塩味の）スナック菓子　epidemiologist／疫学者　the Division for Heart Disease and Stroke Prevention／心臓病及び心臓発作予防部門　contribute A to B／AをBに与える　up to ～／（最大）～まで　the U.S. Food and Drug Administration (FDA)／アメリカ食品医薬品局　recommended daily allowance／一日当たりの推奨栄養所要量　according to ～／～によれば　be full of ～／～でいっぱいの　nutrition label／栄養表示　make a comparison／比較する

comparisons, try to choose lower sodium options, be sure to eat more fresh fruits, vegetables and meats and cook more at home because that way you have more control over the amount of sodium."

According to the agency's guidelines, individual foods should contain no more than 480 milligrams of sodium and prepared meals, including pasta dishes and sandwiches, should not be in excess of 600 milligrams of salt.

The daily allowance for healthy adults is 2,300 milligrams or a teaspoon of salt.

The FDA says people with heart disease, high blood pressure and kidney disease should limit their salt intake to 1,500 milligrams or less per day.

The study on salt content in packaged grocery items is published in the journal *Preventing Chronic Disease*.

Notes:
option／選択肢　be sure to ～／必ず～する　agency／官庁　individual／個々の　no more than ～／たった～　prepared meal／調理食品　limit A to B／AをBに制限する　less／より少ない　on ～／～に関する

練習問題

A 本文の内容に合うように，各英文の（ ）内に入る最も適切な語句をそれぞれ1つずつ選びなさい。

1. The WHO says high blood pressure, which leads to many deaths or permanent disabilities, affects (ten billion / one billion / one hundred million) people worldwide.
2. According to many research studies, we can lower the risk of stroke and related illnesses by (reducing / keeping / increasing) salt or sodium intake.
3. People in developed countries consume about (ten / fifteen / twenty) times more salt than they need.
4. MacGregor insists lowering salt intake and increasing (sugar / potassium / sodium) can help us reduce the risk of hypertension.
5. The CDC found that more than (one-third / half / two-thirds) of all packaged grocery items in the United States contain levels of salt in excess of government recommendations.

B 音声を聴いて，次の英文の（ ）内に適語を記入しなさい。　track 67〜71

1. Carbohydrates, fats, and proteins （　　　）（　　　）（　　　） the body for use as fuel.
2. People with diabetes need to be more aware of what they eat, in order to （　　　）（　　　）（　　　）（　　　）.
3. In order to cure arthritis completely, Western medicine （　　　）（　　　）（　　　） traditional Chinese medicine would be of great help.
4. It is said that women （　　　）（　　　）（　　　）（　　　） suffer from gout.
5. He slept （　　　）（　　　）（　　　） 3 hours last night.

C 和文に合うように，（ ）内の語句を並べかえて英文をつくりなさい。

1. もし人生をやり直すチャンスがあったとしたら，医者になっているでしょう。
   (a chance, again, to, would, had, if, I, I, a, start, be, doctor, my life, medical).

2. その患者は，手術後3日もしないうちに退院した。
　(after, left, the patient, less, days, three, than, surgery, the hospital).

3. 肥満は食習慣と繋がっている。
　(with, habits, obesity, linked, dietary, is).

4. 政府は社会保障制度に毎年約30兆円を支出しているといわれている。
　(spends, the government, is, on, that, every, about, it, 30, welfare, said, year, programs, yen, trillion).

5. 医師からアルコールは一日二杯に制限するようにいわれた。
　(a, told, two, to, to, the doctor, alcohol, of, me, the amount, intake, limit, glasses, day).

D 次の英語に相当する日本語を下から選び，記号で答えなさい。

1. hypertension　　　(　　)　　2. sodium　　　(　　)
3. intake　　　(　　)　　4. kidney failure　　　(　　)
5. dietary potassium　　　(　　)　　6. processed food　　　(　　)
7. high sugar content　　　(　　)　　8. risk factor　　　(　　)
9. nutrition label　　　(　　)　　10. daily allowance　　　(　　)

　　a. 一日当たりの摂取量　　b. 栄養表示　　c. 加工食品
　　d. 危険因子　　e. 高血圧　　f. 高糖度
　　g. 食事性カリウム　　h. 腎不全　　i. 摂取
　　j. ナトリウム

Unit 12

伝統医療と現代医学の統合

Do you know what traditional and complementary/alternative medicines are? WHO says:

Traditional medicine (TM) refers to the knowledge, skills and practices based on the theories, beliefs and experiences indigenous to different cultures, used in the maintenance of health and in the prevention, diagnosis, improvement or treatment of physical and mental illness. Traditional medicine covers a wide variety of therapies and practices which vary from country to country and region to region. In some countries, it is referred to as 'alternative' or 'complementary' medicine (CAM).

Traditional medicine has been used for thousands of years with great contributions made by practitioners to human health, particularly as primary health care providers at the community level. TM/CAM has maintained its popularity worldwide. Since the 1990s its use has surged in many developed and developing countries.

(WHO ホームページ「Health topics」より)

Americans Turn to Complementary, Alternative Medicine for Pain Relief
Voice of America, November 2, 2009

Complementary and alternative medical practices - which include health products and therapies that aren't generally considered part of conventional medicine - are frequently a part of Americans' health care regimens. That's the finding of a new survey released this month by the National Center for Complementary and Alternative Medicine (NCCAM), which is part of the U.S. National Institutes of Health.

Notes:

traditional medicine／伝統医療　complementary/alternative medicine／補完代替医療(通称CAM)　WHO／世界保健機関(the World Health Organization)　refer to ～／～を表す　practice／実践　based on ～／～に基づく　indigenous to ～／～に固有の　prevention／予防　diagnosis／診断　treatment／治療　a wide variety of ～／種々さまざまな～　vary from A to A／Aによって異なる　thousands of ～／何千もの～　practitioner／開業医　primary health care／一次診療　surge／急増する　conventional／従来の，一般に行われている (conventional medicineは西洋医学のこと)　health care regimen／養生法　survey／調査　release／公表する　the National Center for Complementary and Alternative Medicine (NCCAM) ／アメリカ国立補完統合衛生センター　the U.S. National Institute of Health (NIH)／アメリカ国立衛生研究所

Thirty-eight percent of American adults are using some form of complementary and alternative medicine, known as CAM, to help with their health.

NCCAM Director Dr. Josephine Briggs says the new survey provides the most current, comprehensive and reliable source of information on Americans' use of unconventional remedies such as medicinal herbs, acupuncture, yoga, meditation, massage and chiropractic or osteopathic manipulation.

Most of these patients, Briggs says, hope to alleviate pain.

"The most common reason why people turn to complementary and alternative medicine in our survey results is chronic back pain - far and away, the leading reason to use complementary and alternative medicine," she says. "Neck pain, joint pain, headache: All these other conditions are also given as common reasons. But chronic back pain is the leading reason, a very common and difficult condition to treat."

As the federal government's lead agency for scientific research into CAM therapies, the center funds hundreds of projects and trials, supports training for researchers and encourages integration of proven CAM therapies into conventional practice.

Another important part of NCCAM's mission is to publicize news and information about complementary and alternative medicine, and promote discussions about it between patients and their health care providers.

Briggs notes, "It is very important that people talk to their physicians and other health care providers about their use of complementary and alternative medicine."

She points to a survey NCCAM helped conduct, which revealed that as many as two-thirds of those who were using complementary and alternative medicine were not telling their doctors about it.

"We think this is a very sizeable concern. A dialogue about complementary and alternative medicine is a very key part of safe and integrated care."

It is so important that NCCAM has launched a national education campaign to encourage doctor-patient dialogue on these unconventional health practices.

Notes:

comprehensive ／包括的な　unconventional remedy ／CAMの治療法　A such as B ／BのようなA　medicinal herb ／薬草　acupuncture ／鍼療法　meditation ／瞑想　chiropractic or osteopathic manipulation ／カイロプラクティックまたは整骨　alleviate ／緩和する，軽減する　chronic ／慢性の　far and away ／断然　leading ／主な　joint ／関節　federal government ／連邦政府　lead agency ／最重要機関　fund ／資金を提供する　hundreds of ～／何百もの～　integration ／統合　proven ／立証された　publicize ／公表する　point to ～／～を示す　conduct ／行う　reveal ／明らかにする　those who ～／～な人々　sizeable ／（かなり）大きい　integrated ／統合した　so ～ that ... ／非常に～なので…　launch ／開始する

WHO Pursuing Update on Global Strategy for Traditional Medicine

Voice of America, November 29, 2012

 track 74

HONG KONG—

The origins of traditional medicine in Asia, Africa and the Americas can be traced back thousands of years. A successful history of traditional disease prevention and treatment has been viewed with skepticism by contemporary scientists. But such views
5 seem to be changing.

The World Health Organization is meeting in Hong Kong as preparations continue to update a global strategy for traditional medicine first outlined in 2001.

One fifth of the world's population is believed to rely on traditional healthcare. According to WHO figures, 119 countries have developed regulatory frameworks for
10 traditional medicine - or TM.

Dr. Zhang Qi is coordinator of the Geneva-based agency's traditional and complementary medicine unit.

"This shows we should recognize the existence and harness the potential of TM [traditional medicine] to contribute to healthcare. We also [need to] ensure the safety,
15 quality and effectiveness of TM for the public," he said.

While contemporary clinical science has tended to be skeptical about traditional medicine, the reality, says Professor Rudolf Bauer, is that more than one-third of so-called "modern" medicines are still derived from plants. Another third are modeled on plant structures.

20 "The future goal could be some kind of integrated medicine using both traditional and Western medicine to select the best [treatments] for patients," he said.

The head of the University of Graz Institute of Pharmaceutical Sciences, Bauer says modern medicine appears to be adopting successful methodologies from its older counterpart.

25 "TM is not usually one drug for millions of people, but individual mixtures of

Notes:

pursue／遂行する，続行する　global strategy／世界戦略　skepticism／疑い，懐疑的な態度　contemporary／現代の　seem to ～／～するように思われる　rely on ～／～を信頼している　according to ～／～によれば　regulatory framework／規制の枠組み　harness／利用する　clinical science／臨床科学　tend to ～／～する傾向がある　be derived from ～／～に由来する　the University of Graz Institute of Pharmaceutical Sciences／グラーツ大学薬学部　appear to ～／～するように見える　adopt／採用する　methodology／方法論　counterpart／対応するもの　millions of ～／何百万もの～

different herbs to best treat single patients. This concept of personalized medicine is a very hot topic in Western medicine, especially in cancer treatment. We realized we need more individualized therapies - and this has been the case in TM for hundreds, even thousands of years," he said.

Most experts agree the adoption of traditional medicine is going to rise. Yale University Professor of Pharmacology Dr. Yung-chi Cheng is at the vanguard of modern medical research, inventing widely-used therapies for diseases including cancer, hepatitis, and HIV.

In 1999, Cheng began exploring the overlap between traditional and contemporary medicine. Recently he and his colleagues licensed a compound - PHY906 - to improve treatment outcomes and help relieve the pain of cancer patients undergoing chemotherapy.

"This formula consists of four herbs using exactly the same composition described 1,800 years ago in a classic Chinese medicine book. I call this 'poly-chemical medicine' because it has multiple chemicals. Today you and I use single-chemical medicines. This paradigm will evolve to become the cornerstone of future medicine," he said.

The future looks healthy for traditional medicine, although investment will be required.

In Hong Kong, where the WHO meeting is taking place, 30 percent of the population already uses traditional treatments.

While the Health Department was not prepared to speak to VOA, the new government of the semi-autonomous Chinese city has reiterated its commitment to make traditional medicine one of "six emerging pillar industries."

As representative for 300 traditional medicine producers of the Chinese Manufacturers' Association, Joseph Lau is not persuaded. He notes the government does not even keep import and export data for the industry.

"I think the government is not doing enough to promote traditional medicine. Over

> **Notes:**
> be the case／真相・事実である　Yale University Professor of Pharmacology／イェール大学薬理学教授　be at vanguard of／〜の陣頭に立つ　hepatitis／肝炎　HIV／ヒト免疫不全ウイルス (human immunodeficiency virus)　compound／混合物　outcome／結果　help 〜／〜するのに役立つ　undergo／受ける，経験する　chemotherapy／化学療法　formula／処方，製法　consist of 〜／〜から成り立っている　poly-chemical medicine／ポリケミカル薬 (Dr. Chengの造語)　chemical／化合物　paradigm／範例　evolve／進化・発展する　cornerstone／土台，必要不可欠のもの　investment／投資　take place／起こる　semi-autonomous／半自治状態　reiterate／繰り返して言う　'six emerging pillar industries'／6本の新たな産業の柱　representative／代表者　persuade／納得させる

the years they have passed several laws to regulate production. As a manufacturer, it makes our life a lot harder. But this is a necessary step we have to go through," he said.

The China Daily newspaper observed in September that more investment is required for Hong Kong to emerge as a regional TM hub and challenge the Japanese and Korean manufacturers that control 90 percent of the market.

While regulatory frameworks are expanding and improving, concerns about TM quality persist. This year, European authorities have issued several warnings on potential contamination of traditional medicines from Hong Kong and China.

Nonetheless, from a clinical perspective, the testing of new medicines is becoming increasingly rigorous and the credibility of traditional medicine increasingly robust, observes Dr. Cheng.

"I am a mainstream scientist. I know what the concerns are. Many people take a rejectionist approach to TM. But nowadays evidence and hard science are coming along - many people are starting to consider the possibilities, and I think the mood is changing," he said.

As the modernization of ancient healthcare practices continues, the World Health Organization expects to implement its forthcoming 10-year global strategy for traditional medicine by 2014.

Notes:

regulate／取り締まる，規制する　go through ～／～を経る，経験する　emerge／出現する，台頭する　hub／中心，拠点　persist／持続する　issue／発する　potential／潜在的な　contamination／汚染　rigorous／厳しい　credibility／信頼性，威信　robust／強固な，断固とした　mainstream／主流の　evidence／証拠，エビデンス　hard science／自然科学　implement／実行する　forthcoming／来たる

練 習 問 題

A 次の英文が，本文の内容と一致する場合にはT，一致しない場合にはFを（ ）内に記入しなさい。

1. （　） TM/CAM has a long history and practitioners of TM/CAM have done a lot for human health in their country, region or culture.
2. （　） More than a third of American adults are using CAM to keep their health.
3. （　） Chronic back pain is the most common reason to use CAM.
4. （　） Doctor-patient dialogue on CAM is very important to provide safe and integrated care.
5. （　） More than a half of modern medicines have nothing to do with plants.
6. （　） Modern medicine needs to learn the concept of personalized medicine from traditional medicine.
7. （　） The warnings on potential contamination of traditional medicines issued by European authorities have lowered the credibility of TM.

B 音声を聴いて，次の英文の（ ）内に適語を記入しなさい。　　　track 75〜79

1. The film is (　　　) (　　　) a real story.
2. Cultures (　　　) (　　　) country (　　　) country.
3. The era of the solar car (　　　) (　　　) be coming soon.
4. The word *juban* (　　　) (　　　) (　　　) Portuguese.
5. (　　　) (　　　) (　　　), the man has lived alone.

C 和文に合うように，（ ）内の語句を並べかえて英文をつくりなさい。

1. その患者は，手術の同意書に署名をするのをためらっている様子だった。
（appeared, for, her operation, hesitate, sign, the consent form, the patient, to, to）.

2. 英国では，失業した若者が数多くいますが，これは日本も同様です。
（a lot, also, and, are, in Japan, in UK, is, of, there, the case, this, young people, unemployed）.

3. 子どもたちは，お祭りの準備を手伝っていた。
   (children, for, helping, prepare, the festival, were).

4. 日本の人口は，194カ国の国籍で構成されている。
   (194 nationalities, consists, Japan, of, of, population, the).

5. 大きな苦難を経験したことのある人は，他人の気持ちに共感できる。
   (can, ever, empathize, gone, great hardship, have, others, people, through, who, with).

D 次の英語に相当する日本語を下から選び，記号で答えなさい。

1. ayurveda (　　) 2. homeopathy (　　)
3. naturopathy (　　) 4. herbal remedy (　　)
5. supplements (　　) 6. Yin Yang (　　)
7. tai chi (　　) 8. noninvasive treatment (　　)
9. aroma therapy (　　) 10. prayer (　　)

> a. 太極拳　　　　b. 栄養補助食品　　c. 陰陽
> d. 同毒療法　　　e. アロマテラピー　　f. アーユルヴェーダ
> g. 薬草療法　　　h. 自然療法　　　　i. 祈り
> j. 非侵襲的治療

Unit 13

卵巣がんとの闘い

Battling Ovarian Cancer: Clara's Story

Voice of America, March 19, 2015

track 80

The Ovarian Cancer National Alliance says almost a quarter of a million women worldwide are diagnosed with ovarian cancer every year. It is a disease that effects women's ovaries, which are part her reproductive system.

Ovarian cancer is sometimes called the silent killer because its symptoms mimic so
5 many other conditions and in many cases the disease is not discovered until the cancer has spread.

For Clara Frenk, 2013 was unlike any other year of her life.

Clara, who is in her 40's, lives in Washington, D.C. She works full time as a TV production specialist for the Voice of America in the nation's bustling capital.

10 However, she learned that the nagging health problems she was experiencing in the early part of 2013 were symptoms of a bigger problem that was proving tough to identify.

Clara couldn't stay awake

"I realized that the first real symptom that I had was extreme exhaustion," she said.
15 "And when I say extreme exhaustion, I'm not saying feeling a little bit sleepy. I mean it was the kind of exhaustion that I could not keep my eyes open. I was falling asleep at my desk."

"At home I couldn't do anything, really. I couldn't lead a productive life because all I wanted to do was sleep and it was causing a tremendous amount of tension in my
20 marriage, so I consulted with a doctor and I was diagnosed with narcolepsy."

The doctor prescribed stimulants that worked for a little while, "but then the

Notes:

ovarian caner／卵巣がん　Ovarian Cancer National Alliance／卵巣がん全米連合　be diagnosed with ～／～と診断される　ovary／卵巣　reproductive system／生殖器系　silent killer／サイレント・キラー（あまり注目されないが，命取りになることが多い隠れた危険因子）　symptom／症状　mimic／よく似る　bustling／騒がしい　nagging／絶えずつきまとう　fall asleep／寝入る　all I want to do is ～／私が望むのはただ～することだけだ　tremendous／ものすごい　narcolepsy／睡眠発作，ナルコレプシー　prescribe／処方する　stimulant／興奮薬，刺激薬　for a little while／しばらくのあいだ

exhaustion would come right back."

Along with battling exhaustion, the area around Clara's abdomen began to swell, so much so that her mother asked if she was expecting a baby. Clara grew depressed.

25 "I tried every kind of diuretic," she said. "I tried every kind of natural remedy. I also started to develop intense pain in my neck and in my shoulders and in my knees to the point where I couldn't crouch down easily so I went to see a rheumatologist thinking maybe I had arthritis or maybe even fibromyalgia."

The doctor detected a minor case of osteoarthritis in her neck in X-rays, but couldn't 30 determine the cause of her swollen abdomen. So he referred Clara to a gastroenterologist.

Searching the internet for the cause

Clara started to develop a brutal gastric reflux problem.

"I couldn't keep anything down," she said. "My esophagus was burning raw because 35 of all the gastric acid that was coming up continuously."

She researched her symptoms on the Internet and she said, "... and all of them pointed to ovarian cancer," said Clara.

Four symptoms - bloating; difficulty eating or feeling full very quickly; abdominal or pelvic pain and needing to go to the bathroom frequently or urgently - frequently occur 40 with women who have ovarian cancer, says Amanda Davis, director of marketing and communications for the Ovarian Cancer National Alliance in Washington D.C.

"Many women will experience those symptoms at one or more times during her life and that doesn't mean that she necessarily has ovarian cancer," she said. "Several of those symptoms [especially] if they are new or unusually persistent, might be a sign 45 that she should see her doctor and get checked out."

A CT scan confirmed Clara's worst fears. It showed malignant tumors on her ovaries. It also showed there were malignancies in the fluid surrounding her abdomen called ascites. This building of fluid had been the source of the swelling in Clara's abdomen,

---

Notes:

along with ～／〜に加えて　abdomen／腹部　be expecting／出産予定である　depressed／うつ病の，抑うつ症状の　diuretic／利尿薬　natural remedy／自然療法　rheumatologist／リウマチ専門医　arthritis／関節炎　fibromyalgia／線維筋痛症　osteoarthritis／変形性関節炎, 骨関節炎　X-ray／X線（写真）　refer A to B／AをBへ紹介する　gastroenterologist／消化器専門医　brutal／厳しい　gastric reflux／胃酸逆流　esophagus／食道　burn raw／ヒリヒリする　because of ～／〜が原因で　gastric acid／胃酸　point to ～／〜の証拠となる，〜の可能性を示す　bloating／膨満　pelvic pain／骨盤痛　not necessarily ～／必ずしも〜とは限らない　CT scan／CTスキャン　malignant／悪性の（benign ＝ 良性の）　tumor／腫瘍　malignancy／悪性, 悪性腫瘍　ascites／腹水（症）

and of the pain and gastric reflux problems.

Clara was referred to an obstetrical gynecologist who performed surgery.

"I had a radical hysterectomy, so everything was removed from the uterus to the fallopian tubes to the ovaries. The doctor also removed what is called the omentum, which is a fatty sheath that protects the abdomen, so that was kind of a thrown-in benefit which is - I had kind of an ad hoc tummy tuck done. And also, my bowel was restructured," she added.

Prior to the surgery, Clara said she went back to the Internet to look up the survival rates of women with her type of ovarian cancer and found they were extremely dire.

Surviving a perfect post-surgical storm

"A diagnosis of ovarian cancer with malignant ascites means that your cancer has been diagnosed at a very late stage. And after the surgery I was diagnosed with stage three C. It was staged after the surgery," said Clara.

"The survival rate is extremely poor," she said. "I think that someone with three-C malignant ascites, the five-year survival rate is less than 30 percent — may even be less than 20. So I was terrified - absolutely terrified. That's the only way to put it."

Despite the grim statistics Clara did receive some good news regarding her cancer. She was told that all of the cancer had been removed and with the proper form of chemotherapy her chances of surviving for five years would dramatically improve.

Clara chose a chemotherapy that was administered to her using a patch. It was also during her months of treatment that she said she learned to enjoy the small comforts of her life.

How a puppy can help

"It was after the chemotherapy was over and my hair started to grow back that I turned to other comforts like my husband," she said. "And we bought a puppy which was very therapeutic. I started experimenting more and more with make-up which is very relaxing and creative and something that I enjoy."

"So, again you just have to take the good news in dribs and drabs and big chunks if

---

Notes:

obstetrical gynecologist／産婦人科医　surgery／手術　radical／根治的な　hysterectomy／子宮摘出術　uterus／子宮　fallopian tube／ファロピアス管　omentum／（腹腔の）網　ad hoc／その場限りの　tummy tuck／腹部形成 (abdominoplasty)　bowel／腸　prior to ～／～より前に　dire／恐ろしい　less than ～／～未満　regarding ～／～に関して　chemotherapy／化学療法　be over／終わる　in dribs and drabs／少しずつ

you can. But just keep on holding on for the next bit of good news," she added.

Clara has been in remission for one year now and her new oncologist said if she stays in remission for six years, the chances are that the cancer will not come back. At present she goes for check-ups every three months to see if the tumors are returning.

"There are a number of risk factors and we are learning about more every day as our knowledge of this disease expands," Amanda Davis said.

"We know that some aspects that can reduce women's risk include things like having been pregnant, giving birth to children and breastfeeding. We also know that not having done those things can increase risks, and that some women have genetic mutations that can drastically increase their chances of getting ovarian cancer," Davis said.

She added that her organization is constantly working to bring awareness to ovarian cancer which includes meeting with leaders on Washington D.C.'s Capitol Hill to advocate for funding for research and education for ovarian cancer.

Davis also emphasized that one of the biggest challenges in raising awareness about ovarian cancer is that women do not think about it until they get it or someone they know has the disease, especially since there are presently no early detection tests.

Clara has no time to lose

In the meantime, Clara says she is spending more time enjoying the small joys of life - having facials and traveling with her husband.

"We all know that life is finite," she said. "But for me, the finish line may have been pushed up quite a bit so there is no time to lose. Now is the time to do what you enjoy doing and to stop putting off the things that you have been putting off. And try to enjoy every day as much as you can. Things that used to bother me a lot don't bother me as much as they used to."

Clara adds that the Internet is a good source of information on ovarian cancer and for support groups, but she warns it should not be used as the sole source of information.

"While the internet is a good resource, it's a good place to find groups to turn to for

Notes:

keep on ～ing／～し続ける　hold on／頑張る　remission／寛解　oncologist／腫瘍専門医　the chances are that ～／たぶん～であろう　at present／現在は　check-up／検査, 健康診断　a number of ～／たくさんの～　pregnant／妊娠した　give birth to ～／～を産む　genetic mutation／遺伝子突然変異　Capitol Hill／米国連邦議会　detection／検出　in the meantime／その間に　spend A（時間）～ing／A（時間）を使って～する　facial／美顔術　now is the time to ～／今こそ～するチャンスだ　put off ～／～を延期する　used to ～／以前は～であった　support group／サポートグループ（共通の悩みや経験を有していて支援しあう人たちのグループ）

105 comfort ... use it as a resource, but don't allow what you see to frighten you to the point that you throw up your hands and say I give up," she said. "Work with your doctor and just keep on fighting."

練習問題

A 本文の内容に合うように，各英文の（　）内に入る最も適切な語句をそれぞれ1つずつ選びなさい。

1. Almost (half of a million / a quarter of a million / a quarter of billion) women worldwide are diagnosed with ovarian cancer every year.
2. The (diuretics / stimulants / antacids) the doctor prescribed worked, but then the exhaustion came right back.
3. Prior to the surgery, Clara went back to the (hospital, library, Internet) to look up the survival rates of women with her type of ovarian cancer.
4. Clara goes for check-ups (every month / every three months / once a year) to see if tumors are returning.
5. Clara is spending more time (surfing the Internet, walking a dog, traveling with her husband).

B 音声を聴いて，次の英文の（　）内に適語を記入しなさい。　track 81〜85

1. He was recently (　　　)(　　　) diabetes.
2. Jack was arrested (　　　)(　　　) nine other men.
3. (　　　)(　　　)(　　　)(　　　), I worked in the Sales Department.
4. She walked slowly (　　　)(　　　) her bad leg.
5. Morgan (　　　)(　　　)(　　　) a healthy baby girl.

C 和文に合うように，（　）内の語句を並べかえて英文をつくりなさい。

1. 死ぬ前に少しだけ楽しめればいい。
   (is, I, fun, to, die, before, want, have, I, all, a little, do).

2. たぶん列車はまだ出発していないだろう。
   (the train, yet, are, hasn't, chances, left, that, the).

3. 今こそ心を開くときだ。
   (to, heart, now, your, the, open, time, is).

4. 今日できることを明日まで延ばすな。
   (tomorrow, do, can, off, what, today, till, put, you, don't).

5. 現在は以前ほどよくは映画を見に行かない。
   (go, now, to, don't, as, the movies, often, I, to, as, used, I).

D 次の英語に相当する日本語を下から選び，記号で答えなさい。

1. ovarian cancer （　）がん
2. gastric cancer （　）がん
3. esophageal cancer （　）がん
4. arthritis （　）炎
5. hepatitis （　）炎
6. bronchitis （　）炎
7. chemotherapy （　）療法
8. physical therapy （　）療法
9. occupational therapy （　）療法
10. gene therapy （　）療法

a. 胃	b. 遺伝子	c. 化学
d. 肝	e. 関節	f. 気管支
g. 作業	h. 食道	i. 物理
j. 卵巣		

Unit 14

"最期のとき"をどう決めるか

> ### A Woman Ends Her Pain, But the Law Just Won't Let Go
> ### Exit International Member's Death Prompts Victoria Police to Suspect Assisted Suicide
>
> The Age, March 24, 2015

🎧 track 86

Dorothy Hookey thought she had everything in place.

The 86-year-old had enrolled her husband Graham into cooking classes to make sure he could look after himself when she was gone. She had emptied the house of useless objects for the local op shop to benefit. And she had obtained her "insurance" – a lethal
5　drug that could gently take her breath away when the time was right.

The long-time member of pro-euthanasia group Exit International also knew that when she decided to take her last dose of medicine, she had to be alone.

As much as she might have wanted the familiar embrace of her husband as she died, getting him involved would only put him at risk of being charged with aiding or
10　abetting a suicide – an offence that carries a maximum penalty of five years' jail.

So when years of intolerable arthritic pain finally took its toll last year, putting her at imminent risk of being hospitalised until the end, Mrs Hookey secretly implemented her final exit strategy.

Notes:

have everything in place ／すべてを整えておく　cooking class ／料理教室　make sure ～／必ず～であるようにする　look after oneself ／自活する　when she was gone ／彼女が亡くなった時（ここでのgoneは「あの世に行ってしまう」「逝く」の意味）　empty ～ of ... ／～から…を取り除いて空にする　op shop (= opportunity shop) ／《豪》慈善のために中古品を売る店 (charity shop)　lethal drug ／致死薬　take one's breath away ／take one's breath awayは通常「(人)をはっとさせる」などの意味であるが，ここでは「～の呼吸を失わせる」つまり「息を引き取らせる」の意味　pro-euthanasia group Exit International ／安楽死擁護団体イグジット・インターナショナル　familiar embrace ／いつもの抱擁　at risk ／危険な状態に　be charged with ～／～で告発(告訴)される　aiding or abetting a suicide ／自殺ほう助　offence ／《豪／英》(= offense) 罪　maximum penalty of five years' jail ／最高懲役5年の刑罰（なお，オーストラリアでは，jailを以前はgoalと綴ることが多かったが，最近はjailと綴ることが多い）　intolerable arthritic pain ／耐えられない関節炎の痛み　take one's toll ／(人)に悪影響(大損害)を与える　imminent ／切迫した，差し迫った　hospitalise ／《豪／英》(= hospitalize) 入院させる　until the end ／亡くなるまで　implement ／(計画など)を実行する　final exit strategy ／最終出口計画（自分の命を自分で終える計画。exitの語を利用しているのは，上記Exit Internationalという団体の支援を得る計画のため）

After saying goodnight to Mr Hookey and two of her four adult children who were staying with them on November 26, Mrs Hookey sat up in her bed and swallowed her fatal drug. It was accompanied by a nip of her favourite wine, which helped her to go to sleep every night.

　"I got up about 3 a.m. and realised her bedroom light was still on," said Mr Hookey. "She was sitting up in bed with a book and I thought she was asleep but when I rubbed her hand, I realised she was cold."

　Fearing she had had a heart attack, Mr Hookey, 85, called an ambulance and woke up his adult children who were instructed to perform CPR until paramedics arrived. It was useless. She was gone.

　The next day, Mr Hookey said he realised there was a suicide note tucked into the corner of her bedside table. After telling the undertaker, the police jumped on it.

　"Within minutes, there were about six policemen and three detectives roaring through the house," he said. "There were forensics, they were photographing and taking things in little bags and they got statements from me and my other two children."

　Ever since, Mr Hookey and his family have been subjected to an increasingly alarming police investigation, and they now fear they may be caught up in the controversy surrounding Philip Nitschke – the founder of Exit International who is being investigated by police and health authorities for helping several people take their lives.

　Mr Hookey said after a police search of his home on the day after his wife's death, more police returned earlier this month to execute a warrant with the words "assist suicide" on it. They took the family's computer and iPad, and tried to find any books that Mrs Hookey might have used to plan her death.

Notes:

adult children／成人した子どもたち（日本語でいう大人になりきれない人（アダルト・チルドレン）とは意味が違う。）　sit up in one's bed／ベッド上で上半身を起こした状態で座る　fatal drug／（85ページのlethal drugと同じ）　a nip／（強いアルコール飲料の）1杯　favourite／favoriteの豪［英］式綴り　realised／realizedの豪［英］式綴り　her bedroom light was still on／彼女のベッドルームの灯りはまだついていた　rub her hand／彼女の手をさする　heart attack／心臓発作　ambulance／救急車　woke up／起こした　be instructed to ～／指示を受けて～する　CPR／心肺蘇生法（＝ cardiopulmonary resuscitation）　paramedic／パラメディック，上級救急救命士　useless／無駄な　suicide note／自殺(死)の際のメモ書き　tuck／挟み込む，押し込む　undertaker／葬儀屋　jump on ～／～にすぐに取りかかる，～に飛びつく　detective／探偵　roar through the house／家にどやどやと押しかける(入り込む)　forensic／科学捜査官　statement／供述　be subjected to ～／～にさらされている　increasingly alarming／ますます不安にさせるような　police investigation／警察による捜査　Philip Nitschke／フィリップ・ニチキ（(1947-) Exit Internationalの創始者のオーストラリア人）　execute／執行する　warrant（＝ warrant of arrest, arrest warrant)／逮捕状　"assist suicide"／「自殺ほう助」

"It's such a kick in the guts. I've been waiting for the sword of Damocles to fall ever since," he said, even though he feels he has done nothing wrong.

40 Mr Hookey said it hurt to be treated like a criminal while he was mourning his wife's death – an end he described as a rational choice made by an independent woman who did not want to die in a hospital or nursing home with no control over what happened to her.

"To me, it's just such a shocking waste of police resources," said Mr Hookey, who is a
45 Justice of the Peace and son of a policeman.

The treasurer of his local Probus club is also angry that his wife felt that she had to be alone when she died, and that even making the sacrifice of dying alone had not protected her family from scrutiny.

"If she had of been able to get in the car and drive somewhere to do it, I don't think
50 this would have happened. But because we were in the house, we're now suspects," he said. "I find that tragic ... and I think it is a dreadful indictment on our social system."

A spokeswoman for Victoria Police would not comment on whether charges would be laid, but said detectives were preparing a report for the coroner.

> **Notes:**
>
> kick in the guts／心にひどくこたえること，落ち込ませる（がっかりさせる）こと　the sword of Damocles／ダモクレスの剣，いつ起こるかもしれぬ危険（王の幸福をうらやんだので，王はダモクレスを王座につかせ，彼の頭上から髪の毛一本で剣をつるし，王位の危険を教えた故事による）　Damocles／ダモクレス（紀元前4世紀シラクサ（Syracuse）の王Dionysiusの廷臣）　even though ～／たとえ～だとしても　rational choice／合理的選択　nursing home／高齢者施設，老人ホーム　Justice of the Peace／治安判事　Probus club／プロバスクラブ（ロータリークラブが，社会奉仕事業の一環として退職者およびセミ退職者のためにつくった親睦団体。Professional Businessmanの略語とラテン語のProbus（誠実）という語をかける）　sacrifice／犠牲　scrutiny／詮索，捜査　had of been／正しくはhad have been（話し言葉を発音通りに表記している）　suspect／容疑者　indictment／《発音注意》欠陥　charge／告発，容疑　coroner／検死官

Voluntary Euthanasia: Knowledge of Father's Plans Protected Family

The Age, March 25, 2015

track 87

My heart aches for the Hookey family, who are now being punished by a cruel and irrational law following the chosen death of their wife and mother ("Family's pain over investigation", 24/3), who acted, as she lovingly believed, in ways to ensure her family was protected from suspicion.

My father died in exactly the same chosen circumstances as Dorothy Hookey. He was in intolerable pain from a number of age-related conditions that were resulting in breathing difficulties, incontinence, constant abdominal pain, arthritis and, most grievously to a formerly voracious reader, loss of vision to the point of legal blindness. For decades, he had told his family he wanted to die in his own way at his own time. At 93, having carefully ordered his affairs and made his plans, he decided his time was up. He died in the evening at home, in his own bed, peacefully, with members of his immediate family nearby.

The only difference between Dorothy Hookey's chosen death and my father's is that we were not subject to terror by a punitive law. Why? In the weeks prior to his death, my father told his three adult children of his plans, in addition to advising his long-time GP. He took the risk that giving us all this information would be ultimately protective; and so it was. And that I next morning called the GP, rather than an ambulance.

The police are only doing their job. It is the law prohibiting an individual choosing the circumstances of their death, and which implies culpability to anyone with knowledge of their plans, that needs urgent and critical review. For the sake of us all, including the police, our politicians must refer proposed law reform to enable choice at the end of life and physician-assisted dying to the Victorian Law Reform Commission

---

Notes:

ache／痛む irrational／不合理な(↔rational, 87ページのrational choice参照) age-related／年齢に起因する result in ～／～という結果となる breathing difficulties／呼吸困難 incontinence／失禁 abdominal pain／腹痛 arthritis／関節炎 grievously／つらく, 苦しく formerly voracious reader／以前本の虫だった人, 熱烈に読書好きだった人 loss of vision／失明 legal blindness／法的に盲目とされる状態 for decades／何十年間 immediate family／肉親 punitive law／刑法 prior to ～／～の前 tell ～ of …／～に…のことを言う(ofの代わりにaboutも使われる) in addition to ～／～に加えて GP／一般開業医(= general practitioner) culpability／有罪 physician-assisted dying／医師のほう助による殺人 the Victorian Law Reform Commission／ビクトリア州法改正委員会

for consideration and recommendations.

Name and address withheld

Nothing civilised about investigation

Congratulations on yesterday's front-page article and Monday's obituary on Terry Pratchett ("Writer's world of comic fantasy sold more than 85 million books", 23/3).

You are supporting the more than 80 per cent of us who think people who wish to end their own lives because of intolerable suffering should be able to do so. There's nothing civilised about the increasingly alarming police investigation to which Dorothy Hookey's family is being subjected. Anyone who saw Pratchett's documentary *Choosing to Die* knows it is possible for a civilised, legal and safeguarded process giving people the right to die to be put in place, if our governments only had the will to do so. When are our elected representatives going to start listening to the vast majority of us on this issue?

Kaye Cole, Princes Hill

Police should charge Nitschke

I offer my condolences to Mr Hookey on the death of his wife. I can understand he is upset with the police involvement. My son also died alone; he took his own life in January last year at the age of 25. He ordered Nembutal through the Exit International site, too. We did not know he was suicidal. The police are involved in your wife's death because it is against the law to assist a person to suicide. The person who should be charged is Philip Nitschke.

Mary Waterman, Arthur's Seat

Notes:

name and address withheld ／氏名及び住所は秘匿　civilised ／お上品な　Monday's obituary on Terry Pratchett ／月曜日の Terry Pratchett の死亡記事（Terry Pratchett は英国の作家で 2015 年 3 月 12 日死去。彼の追悼記事として "Writer's world of comic fantasy sold more than 85 million books" が 3 月 23 日の月曜日に掲載された）　Terry Pratchett ／テリー・プラチェット（1948-2015）（英国の SF 作家・ファンタジー作家，作品には *Terry Pratchett: Choosing to Die* という自ら死を選択することをテーマとしたものもあり，投稿者は投稿文中，この作品に言及している。ちなみにこのドキュメンタリー番組はインターネットの動画サイトでの視聴が可能である）　because of 〜／〜が原因で　put in place ／（あるべき場所に）置かれる　elected representative ／選挙で選ばれた代表（議員のこと）　vast majority ／大多数　condolences ／お悔やみ　upset ／気が動転して　take one's own life ／自らの命を奪う　Nembutal ／ネンブタール（鎮静・催眠薬 pentobarbital sodium の商品名）　suicidal ／自殺願望のある

Is this what Victorians want?

The police are just doing their job – enforcing Victorian law. The law allows a person to take their life by hanging, suffocation and so on, but not by peaceful means. Is this a law we all voted for? Is this a situation we want – that family members have to make sure that when their suffering is intolerable and untreatable and they've chosen to go, that they leave their home, as well as dying alone?

Janine Truter, The Basin

練 習 問 題

A 本文の内容に合うように，各英文の（　）内に入る最も適切な語句をそれぞれ1つずつ選びなさい。

1. Fearing she had had a heart attack, Mr Hookey, 85, called an (ambulatory / abduction / ambulance).
2. His adult children were instructed to perform CPR until (paramounts / paramedics / parasites) arrived.
3. There were (forensics / forestry / forerunners), photographing and taking things in a little bags.
4. I find that (comical / tragic / heroic) I think it is a dreadful indictment on our social system.
5. I offer my (condolences / conductivity / condemnation) to Mr Hookey on the death of his wife.

B 音声を聴いて，次の英文の（　）内に適語を記入しなさい。　　track 88〜92

1. The 86-year-old had enrolled her husband Graham into cooking classes (　　　)(　　　)(　　　) he could look after himself when she was gone.
2. Mrs Hookey (　　　)(　　　) her final exit strategy.
3. Mrs Hookey (　　　)(　　　)(　　　)(　　　)(　　　) and swallowed her fatal drug.
4. They tried to find any books that Mrs Hookey (　　　)(　　　)(　　　) to plan her death.
5. We did not know he was (　　　).

C 和文に合うように，（　）内の語句を並べかえて英文をつくりなさい。

1. 彼女が最後の一服の薬品を飲むと決めた時は，一人でいなくてはならなかった。
 (be alone, when, of medicine, had to, decided to, she, she, her last, take, dose).

2. 私は午前3時頃起き，彼女のベッドルームの明かりはまだついていることを認識しました。
 (I, and, got up, was, realised, light, still, about 3 am, on, her bedroom).

Unit 14　91

3. それは，そんなに心にひどく答えたことでした。
   (is, kick, it, the, a, such, guts, in).

4. 彼は，何も悪いことをしていないと感じています。
   (has, wrong, nothing, he, he, done, feels).

5. 私は，それは私たちの社会システムのひどい欠陥だと思います。
   (think, social system, I, is, dreadful indictment, it, a, on, our).

D 次の英語に相当する日本語を下から選び，記号で答えなさい。

1. euthanasia (　　　)
2. aiding a suicide または abetting a suicide (　　　)
3. arthritis (　　　)
4. arthritic pain (　　　)
5. intolerable pain (　　　)
6. age-related (　　　)
7. nursing home (　　　)
8. breathing difficulties (　　　)
9. incontinence (　　　)
10. abdominal pain (　　　)
11. blindness (　　　)
12. GP (　　　)

a. 安楽死	b. 一般開業医	c. 関節炎の痛み
d. 高齢者施設	e. 呼吸困難	f. 自殺ほう助
g. 耐えられない痛み	h. 尿失禁	i. 年齢に起因する
j. 関節炎	k. 腹痛	l. 盲目

Unit 15
「老年植民地主義」または「姥捨て貿易」か?

Some with Alzheimer's Find Care in Far-Off Nations

The Japan News, January 18, 2014　　Associated Press

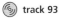 track 93

CHIANG MAI, Thailand —

Residents of this facility for people with Alzheimer's disease toss around a yellow ball and laugh under a cascade of water with their caregivers, in a swimming pool ringed by palm trees and wind chimes. Susanna Kuratli, once a painter of delicate oils, swims a lap
5　and smiles.

Watching is her husband, Ulrich, who has a heart-rending decision: to leave his wife of 41 years in this facility 9,000 kilometers (5,600 miles) from home, or to bring her back to Switzerland.

Their homeland treats the elderly as well as any nation on earth, but Ulrich Kuratli
10　says the care here in northern Thailand is not only less expensive but more personal. In Switzerland, "You have a cold, old lady who gives you pills and tells you to go to bed," he says.

Kuratli and his three grown children have given themselves six months to decide while the retired software developer lives alongside his 65-year-old wife in Baan
15　Kamlangchay—"Home for Care from the Heart." Patients live in individual houses within a Thai community, are taken to local markets, temples and restaurants, each with

Notes:

Chiang Mai／チエンマイ(タイ北西部にあるミャンマーと国境を接する県およびその中心都市)　people with Alzheimer's disease／アルツハイマーの方々（Alzheimer's disease peopleやAlzheimer's disease patientのようには表現せず, people with Alzheimer's diseaseというのがよいとされる。このような考えをpeople-first languageとよび, 当事者の尊厳を尊重する言い方であるとされる）　cascade／滝　caregiver／介護者　ringed by ～／～で囲まれた　palm tree／ヤシの木　wind chime／風鈴　a lap／一周　heart-rending／胸を引き裂くような, 悲痛な　wife of 41 years／41年連れ添った妻　as well as ～／～と同様　not only A but B／Aだけでなく Bも　personal／ひとりひとりに合わせた　You have a cold, old lady who gives you pills and tells you to go to bed／あなたが風邪をひく, あなたに薬をくれる老女あなたに寝ろという(英語が母語ではない(ドイツ語話者)スイス人なので, やや不自然な英語になっている)　grown children／成人した子供たち(＝adult children, p.86)　retired／退職した　software developer／ソフトウェア開発者　Baan Kamlangchay／バーン・カムランチャイ(タイ語で「心からのケアを行う施設(Home for Care from the Heart)」の意味の名称をもつドイツ語話者専門の認知症患者受け入れ施設)　local market／地元の市場(マーケット)

three caretakers working in rotation to provide personal around-the-clock care. The monthly $3,800 cost is a third of what basic institutional care would come to in Switzerland.

Kuratli is not yet sure how he'll care for Susanna, who used to produce a popular annual calendar of her paintings. But he's leaning toward keeping her in Thailand, possibly for the rest of her life.

"Sometimes I am jealous. My wife won't take my hand but when her Thai carer takes it, she is calm. She seems to be happy," he says. "When she sees me she starts to cry. Maybe she remembers how we were and understands, but can no longer find the words."

Spouses and relatives in Western nations are increasingly confronting Kuratli's dilemma as the number of Alzheimer's patients and costs rise, and the supply of qualified nurses and facilities struggles to keep up. Faraway countries are offering cheaper, and to some minds better, care for those suffering from the irreversible loss of memory.

The nascent trend is unnerving to some experts who say uprooting people with Alzheimer's will add to their sense of displacement and anxiety, though others say quality of care is more important than location. There's also some general uneasiness over the idea of sending ailing elderly people abroad: The German press has branded it "gerontological colonialism."

Germany is already sending several thousand sufferers, as well as the aged and otherwise ill, to Eastern Europe, Spain, Greece and Ukraine. Patients are even moving from Switzerland, which was ranked No. 1 in health care for the elderly this year in an index compiled by the elderly advocacy group HelpAge International and the U.N.

Notes:

caretaker／介護者（caregiver）　working in rotation／ローテンション勤務の　around-the-clock care／24時間体制の介護　institutional care／施設ケア　come to ～／（値段・金額など）が～になる　used to ～／かつては～していた　produce a popular annual calendar of her paintings／自分自身の絵で毎年有名なカレンダーをつくる（ちなみに彼女のカレンダーはインターネットで入手可能）　lean toward ～／～に（気持ちが）傾く　for the rest of one's life／人生の残りの期間、死ぬまで　Thai／タイ人の　carer／介護人　no longer ～／もはや～でない　spouse／配偶者　confront／直面する　dilemma／ジレンマ　qualified nurses and facilities／資格のある看護師および施設　struggle to keep up／現状維持がやっとである　faraway／遠い　to some minds／ある人たちにとっては　suffer from ～／～にかかる、～に苦しむ　irreversible loss of memory／回復不能の記憶喪失　nascent／新しい、新規の　unnerving／不安にさせる　uproot ～／（人）をこれまで住んでいた土地から離れさせる　add to ～／～を増す　sense of displacement／疎外感、場違いな気持ち　anxiety／不安感　general uneasiness／一般的心配（懸念）　ailing／病弱な　"gerontological colonialism"／「老年植民地主義」　otherwise ill／ほかの傷病をもつ人たち　compile／編集する　elderly advocacy group／高齢者権利擁護団体　HelpAge International／ヘルプエイジ・インターナショナル（高齢者の権利を擁護する国際団体、1983年設立）

Population Fund.

The Philippines is offering Americans care for $1,500 to $3,500 a month—as compared to $6,900 the American Elder Care Research Organization says is the average monthly bill for a private room in a skilled nursing US facility. About 100 Americans are currently seeking care in the Philippines but more facilities are being built and a marketing campaign will be launched in 2014, says J.J. Reyes, who is planning a retirement community near Manila.

Facilities in Thailand also are preparing to attract more Alzheimer's sufferers. In Chiang Mai, a pleasant city ringed by mountains, Baan Kamlangchay will be followed by a $10 million, holiday-like home scheduled to open before mid-2014. Also on the way is a small Alzheimer's unit within a retirement community set on the grounds of a former four-star resort. With Thailand seeking to strengthen its already leading position as a medical tourism and retirement destination, similar projects are likely.

The number of people over 60 worldwide is set to more than triple between 2000 and 2050 to 2 billion, according to the World Health Organization. And more are opting for retirement in lower-cost countries.

"Medical tourism" has become a booming industry, with roughly 8 million people a year seeking treatment abroad, according to the group Patients Without Borders.

The UK-based Alzheimer's Disease International says there are more than 44 million Alzheimer's patients globally, and the figure is projected to triple to 135 million by 2050. The Alzheimer's Association estimates that in the United States alone, the disease will cost $203 billion this year and soar to $1.2 trillion by 2050.

The pioneering Baan Kamlangchay was established by Martin Woodtli, a Swiss who

Notes:

the U.N. Population Fund／国連人口基金（国連内の人口的分野を中心的に司る機関，前身が1967年に設立された） the American Elder Care Research Organization／アメリカ高齢ケア研究機関（米国内の高齢ケア専門研究機関） retirement community／退職者コミュニティ（退職した後に，それまでの住宅及び土地を売却するなどして，移り住む退職者専用のコミュニティ（自治体組織）。通常，健全な時に入居し，介護や医療が必要になってもコミュニティ内で生活できるようになっている。） Alzheimer's sufferer／アルツハイマー病患者　also on the way is ～／さらに開業準備中なのは～です（～ is also on the wayが倒置されている）　Alzheimer's unit／アルツハイマー病患者用ユニット　four-star resort／四つ星リゾート地，四つ星リゾート施設　medical tourism／メディカル・ツーリズム（医療を求めて，（とくに外国に）行くこと）　retirement destination／退職後の移住先　according to ～／～によると　the World Health Organization／世界保健機関　lower-cost country／コストがかからない国　booming industry／急速に発展している産業　Patients Without Borders／国境なき患者団（外国で医療を受ける患者たちのための団体）　Alzheimer's Disease International／国際アルツハイマー病協会（アルツハイマー病の患者及びその家族のための国際組織）　globally／世界中で　project／見積もる　the Alzheimer's Association／アルツハイマー協会　pioneering／先駆的な

spent four years in Thailand with the aid group Doctors Without Borders before returning home to care for his Alzheimer's diagnosed mother.

Wanting to return to Thailand and knowing that Thais traditionally regard the elderly with great respect, he brought his mother to Chiang Mai, where she became the home's first "guest." Woodtli never uses the word "patient."

Over the next 10 years, the 52-year-old psychologist and social worker purchased or rented eight two-story houses where 13 Swiss and German patients now reside. Two people normally share the modest but well-kept, fully furnished houses, each sleeping in a separate bedroom along with their caretaker.

Breakfast and lunch are eaten together at another residence where Woodtli, his wife and son live. On most afternoons, the group gathers at a private, walled park to swim, snack and relax on deck chairs. Regular outside activities are organized because he believes these stimuli may help delay degeneration.

"Movement is important. Tensions are also relieved if they have freedom to move. Our carers allow our guests a lot of space as long as it does not pose a danger to them," he says. "In Switzerland we don't have opportunity for such care."

He says his guests "cannot explain it, but I think they feel part of a family, a community, and that is very important."

Yet Woodtli says he has received criticism about "the Swiss starting to export their social problems."

The German press has recently described shifting the aged and ailing abroad as "grandmother export."

Sabine Jansen, head of Germany's Alzheimer Society, says that while some with Alzheimer's may adjust to an alien place, most find it difficult because they live in a world of earlier memories.

Notes:

Doctors Without Borders／国境なき医師団（紛争地域や貧困地域に医療を提供する慈善団体。フランス語ではMédecins Sans Frontières）　Alzheimer's diagnosed／アルツハイマー病の診断を受けた　regard ~ with great respect／~を大きな敬意をもって敬う　psychologist and social worker／心理学者でもありソーシャルワーカーでもある人　fully furnished house／家具などがすべて備え付けられている家　along with ~／~と一緒に　on most afternoons／ほとんどの午後には（in the afternoon（午後に）という場合にはinの前置詞を使うが，afternoon(s)にmostと修飾語がつくので，onとなる。(on the afternoon of October 11 = 10月11日の午後に）　walled park／壁で囲まれた公園　snack／おやつを食べる　deck chair／デッキチェア（ズック布張り折りたたみ式の椅子）　outside activity／屋外活動　stimuli／（stimulusの複数形）刺激　degeneration／退化，老化　tension／緊張感　relieve／緩和させる　as long as ~／~な限りは　criticism／批判，非難　"grandmother export"／「姥捨て貿易」　Germany's Alzheimer Society／ドイツのアルツハイマー協会　alien place／見知らぬ場所，外国の地　earlier memories／以前の記憶

"People with dementia should stay in their familiar environment as long as possible. They are better oriented in their own living places and communities," she says. "Friends, family members, neighbors can visit them. Also because of language and cultural reasons, it is best for most to stay in their home country."

Angela Lunde of the US-based Mayo Clinic says that generally the afflicted do better in a familiar environment, but over time, even those with advanced stages of the disease can adjust well. "I think a positive transition has less to do with the move itself and more with the way in which the staff and new environment accommodates the person living with dementia," she says.

Woodtli agrees that moving to a country like Thailand is not the answer for everyone with Alzheimer's, but those who have traveled widely and are accustomed to change can probably adapt.

"One of our guests sometimes wakes up in the morning and says, 'Where am I?' But she would do the same if she was in a care center in Switzerland," he says. "And they take their past with them. One guest thinks she is in a schoolhouse at Lake Lucerne."

Those who end up staying at a facility being built in the outlying Chiang Mai district of Doi Saket will have amenities that would be tough for its European counterparts to match, including a clubhouse with a massage room and beauty parlor, a restaurant, Swiss bakery and pavilions with soaring ceilings and skylights.

"The idea is that this is a resort, not a hospital," says Marc H. Dumur, a veteran hotelier who will manage the Swiss-owned, 3.5-hectare (8.7-acre) facility built amid orchards and groves of teak. Going up are 72 patient rooms in six spacious pavilions, plus villas for visiting family members. Around-the-clock care will be provided by a staff of 150, including a Swiss head nurse and at least one licensed Thai nurse for each pavilion.

These patient-to-carer ratios reflect the costs in a developing country like Thailand

Notes:

people with dementia／認知症の人たち　better oriented／よりよく適合した　because of ~／~が原因で　Mayo Clinic／メイヨー・クリニック（アメリカ合衆国ミネソタ州ロチェスター市に本部を置く総合病院）　the afflicted／病人　over time／時間をかければ　those with advanced stages of the disease／その病気の進行がかなり進んだ人たち　has less to do with ~ more with ...／~との関連はより少なく、…との関連はより多い　those who have traveled widely／広く旅をしてきた人々　be accustomed to ~／~に慣れている　schoolhouse／校舎　Lake Lucerne／ルツェルン湖（スイスの湖）　outlying／辺ぴな、中心から離れた　Doi Saket／ドーイ・サケット（チエンマイ県にある郡）　amenities／生活を快適にするもの（施設、環境）　beauty parlor／美容室　pavilion／病棟　skylight／天窓　hotelier／ホテル経営者　grove／小さい林　teak／チーク　villa／別荘　head nurse／看護師長　at least／少なくとも　patient-to-carer ratio／患者対介護者の比率

and the West. A licensed Thai nurse earns less than $700 a month, compared to about $7,000 for one in Switzerland, where care centers will have one nurse responsible for 10 patients.

Care at the Doi Saket home will cost $6,000 a month, roughly what a mid-level employee in Switzerland would receive as a pension, Dumur says.

A number of European countries have generous national health insurance, but these generally do not cover treatment abroad. Kuratli says the Swiss government would cover two-thirds of the bill for his wife's care if she stays in Switzerland, but since high-end private clinics there can cost $15,000 or more per month, he could still end up paying more there than he would in Thailand.

British businessman Peter Brown has turned a bankrupt resort into the Care Resort Chiang Mai. Residents will live in five-room units, watched over by nurses 24 hours a day, and walk out into extensive, landscaped grounds, with a thousand trees and a lake, set in a tranquil area at the foot of mountains.

"In Europe they tend to follow a lock-up system. They know what should be done but they just don't have the staff to do it—to take patients to visit gardens, to give them some freedom," Brown says. "And the carers tend to come from the lower end of the nursing system. They often don't have the desire to work with Alzheimer's patients or an affinity with them."

Woodtli agrees that it is crucial "for the patients to be together with their carers, to know and trust." He says Thai caregivers like those at Baan Kamlangchay are generally more emotionally and physically engaged with their charges.

At the swimming pool, Madeleine Buchmeier snaps photos and laughs as she watches a caregiver take her smiling husband's hands to twirl around together in a dance out of childhood.

"It's a miracle," she says. Geri used to bang his head against the walls of a care facility in Switzerland, she says, "as if he wanted to do something, get somewhere."

He would sink when entering water. In the three weeks since they arrived, he has

---

Notes:

less than ～／～未満　mid-level employee／平均的な従業員(サラリーマン)　pension／年金　a number of ～／多くの～　national health insurance／国民健康保険　high-end／高級な，上流向けの　end up ～ing／～することになる　a bankrupt resort／倒産したリゾート施設　extensive／広大な　landscaped／景色のよい　at the foot of ～／～のふもとの　tend to ～／～する傾向がある　lock-up／施錠式　the lower end of the nursing system／看護システムの下層　affinity／好み，好きなこと　charge／委託された人（ここでは患者のこと）　snap a photo／写真を撮る　twirl around／くるくる回る　dance out of childhood／子ども時代からのダンス　bang one's head against the wall／壁に頭を打ちつける　as if ～／まるで～のように

calmed down and can swim again, all while his medicine is being sharply reduced.

Like Kuratli, Buchmeier is deciding whether her 64-year-old husband should stay or
go back to Switzerland. Once a Ford Motor Co. employee who spoke four languages, he
now mutters largely disjointed sentences but appears to recognize his wife.

Nearby, Manfred Schlaupitz, a former Daimler-Benz engineer in his 70s, lies back in
a deck chair, cradling a stuffed toy lamb. His caregiver, Kanokkan Tasa, sits on the grass
beside him, gently massaging his legs and tickling his chin. She has been with him for
six years, eight hours a day and earlier cared for Woodtli's mother.

"If you think of it as a job it's very difficult," she says, "but if it comes from the heart,
it is easy."

She came to the home with no formal nursing training.

"I felt pity for them and asked myself, 'If I was stricken with Alzheimer's, how would
I want to be cared for?'" she said.

The 32-year-old woman communicates in Thai, German, English and her native
tribal language but most importantly, she says, through eye and physical contact and
displays of emotion.

Like a number of Alzheimer's victims, Schlaupitz responds well to music. Sometimes
they sing one of his favorite songs: "Yesterday."

Notes:

calm down／落ち付く　Ford Motor Co.／フォード自動車会社　disjointed／支離滅裂な　Daimler-Benz engineer／ダイムラー＝ベンツ社のエンジニア　a stuffed toy lamb／子ヒツジのぬいぐるみ　be stricken with Alzheimer's／アルツハイマー病に襲われる　tribal language／部族語　"Yesterday"／「イエスタデイ」(ビートルズ(the Beatles)のヒットソング，1965年発表)

練習問題

A 本文の内容に合うように，各英文の（　）内に入る最も適切な語句をそれぞれ1つずつ選びなさい。

1. The monthly $3,800 cost is (a half / a third / a fourth) of what basic institutional care would come to in Switzerland.
2. Faraway countries are offering cheaper care for those (recovering from / resulting from / suffering from) the irreversible loss of memory.
3. (Quality / Amount / Quantity) of care is more important than location.
4. The number of people over 60 worldwide is set to more than (half / double / triple) between 2000 and 2050 to 2 billion, according to the World Health Organization.

B 音声を聴いて，次の英文の（　）内に適語を記入しなさい。　　track 94～98

1. Their homeland (　　　) the (　　　　) as well as any nation on Earth.
2. Thailand is (　　　) (　　　) less expensive (　　　) more personal.
3. There's some general (　　　　) over the idea of sending (　　　　) elderly people abroad.
4. (　　　) (　　　) has become a booming industry.
5. Regular (　　　　) (　　　　) are organized.

C 和文に合うように，（　）内の語句を並べかえて英文をつくりなさい。

1. 日本の施設はより多くの外国人観光客をひきつけようと準備しています。
  (Japan, attract, foreign, facilities, are, tourists, more, in, to, preparing).

2. もし彼らが動く自由があれば，緊張も緩和されます。
  (move, also, are, have, they, if, to, tensions, relieved, freedom).

3. 認知症の人は，できるだけ長くよく知っている環境にとどまるべきです。
  (with, should stay in, long, familiar environment, dementia, people, their, as, as, possible).

4. 時間をかければ，病気がかなり進行している人たちでもよく適応することができます。
   (advanced stages, well, over time, of the disease, can, even, with, those, adjust).

5. 広く旅をしてきたり，変化に慣れていたりする人たちはおそらく適応できます。
   (who, those, adapt, can, change, and, probably, accustomed to, have traveled widely, are).

D 次の英語に相当する日本語を下から選び，記号で答えなさい。
1. Alzheimer's disease （　）
2. dementia （　）
3. loss of memory （　）
4. anxiety （　）
5. gerontological （　）
6. degeneration （　）
7. retirement community （　）
8. medical tourism （　）
9. caregiver, caretaker, carer （　）

a. アルツハイマー病	b. 介護士	c. 記憶喪失
d. 退職者コミュニティ	e. 認知症	f. 不安感
g. メディカルツーリズム	h. 老化，退化	i. 老年学の

編著者紹介

田中　芳文
（たなか　よしふみ）
　1985 年　岡山大学大学院教育学研究科（英語教育専攻）修了
　現　在　島根県立大学人間文化学部教授

NDC 490　　109p　　26cm

英文ニュースで学ぶ　健康とライフスタイル
（えいぶん）　　（まな）　　（けんこう）

2016 年 9 月 14 日　第 1 刷発行
2022 年 1 月 21 日　第 2 刷発行

編著者　田中芳文
発行者　髙橋明男
発行所　株式会社　講談社
　　　　〒112-8001　東京都文京区音羽 2-12-21
　　　　　　販　売　(03) 5395-4415
　　　　　　業　務　(03) 5395-3615

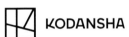

編　集　株式会社　講談社サイエンティフィク
　　　　代表　堀越俊一
　　　　〒162-0825　東京都新宿区神楽坂 2-14　ノービィビル
　　　　　　編　集　(03) 3235-3701
印刷所　豊国印刷株式会社
製本所　株式会社国宝社

落丁本・乱丁本は，購入書店名を明記のうえ，講談社業務宛にお送りください．送料小社負担にてお取替えいたします．なお，この本の内容についてのお問い合わせは，講談社サイエンティフィク宛にお願いいたします．定価はカバーに表示してあります．
© Yoshifumi Tanaka, 2016
本書のコピー，スキャン，デジタル化等の無断複製は著作権法上での例外を除き禁じられています．本書を代行業者等の第三者に依頼してスキャンやデジタル化することはたとえ個人や家庭内の利用でも著作権法違反です．

[JCOPY]〈(社)出版者著作権管理機構委託出版物〉
複写される場合は，その都度事前に(社)出版者著作権管理機構（電話 03-5244-5088，FAX 03-5244-5089, e-mail: info@jcopy.or.jp）の許諾を得てください．

Printed in Japan
ISBN978-4-06-155629-4

やさしい英語ニュースで学ぶ 現代社会と健康
田中 芳文・編著
B5・110頁・定価2,640円（税込）
健康・医療・生活のニュースでトレーニングする英語教科書。一般向け記事なので、現代社会とのつながりを意識しながらスラスラ読める。
ISBN 978-4-06-155633-1

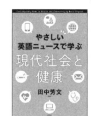

英文ニュースで学ぶ 健康とライフスタイル
田中 芳文・編著
B5・112頁・定価2,860円（税込）
医療や健康の話題を扱ったニュース記事で英語リーディング能力をレベルアップ！ 一般人向けの記事だから、出てくる用語は一般常識レベルで、文章も読みやすい。看護系や健康栄養系の学生のための新しい英語トレーニング！
ISBN 978-4-06-155629-4

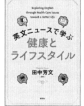

ニュースで読む医療英語　CD付き
川越 栄子・編著
森 茂／田中 芳文／名木田 恵理子／大下 晴美・著
B5・112頁・定価3,080円（税込）
医療・看護のためのやさしい英語テキスト。一般向けのわかりやすい医療ニュースを題材に、入門レベルの読者でもすらすら読める。ネイティブ読み上げCD付きでリスニングもバッチリ！
ISBN 978-4-06-156310-0

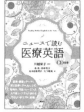

やさしい栄養英語
田中 芳文・編著
中里 菜穂子／松浦 加寿子・著
B5・64頁・定価1,980円（税込）
英語の栄養学読み物を題材にした教科書。一般向けの読み物だから、簡単な英文でスラスラ読める。栄養学の基礎も身について一石二鳥！
用語説明も充実しているので、辞書をひく必要なし。英文の長さや問題の量、本全体のページ数に至るまで、スッキリ学べる手ごろな分量。
ISBN 978-4-06-513414-6

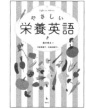

はじめての栄養英語
えっ、Dietって、やせるって意味じゃないの？
栄養士の私はDietitianなんだ！
美味しく学べる英語のスキル
清水 雅子・著
B5・112頁・定価1,980円（税込）
やさしい英文で初学者でも栄養英語に親しめるよう工夫されたテキスト。栄養素、代謝、解剖生理、消化吸収、食品添加物、食物アレルギーなどを、やさしく短い英文でとりあげた。
ISBN 978-4-06-155613-3

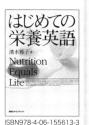

はじめての臨床栄養英語
清水 雅子／J. パトリック・バロン・著
B5・128頁・定価2,530円（税込）
栄養管理を必要とする疾患を中心に、平易な英文で、組織・器官の名称、病気の概要、診断基準、食事療法、薬物療法を学ぶ、これまでにない教科書。病院臨地実習やゼミで必須となる基本英語を集約。大学院受験にも役立つ1冊。
ISBN 978-4-06-155621-8

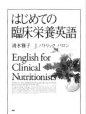

Let's Study English! Health and Nutrition 英語で読む健康と栄養
横尾 信男・編著
A5・96頁・定価1,650円（税込）
栄養系学生のための教養課程英語テキスト。健康な食生活に必要な知識（栄養素やその摂取法、病気にならない食生活・エクササイズ、酒やタバコの害、食中毒、ストレス解消など）を幅広く学べるように編集。
ISBN 978-4-06-153951-8

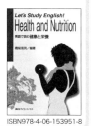

耳から学ぶ 楽しいナース英語　CD付き
中西 睦子・監修　野口 ジュディー／川越 栄子／仁平 雅子・著
B5・112頁・定価3,740円（税込）
CDを聞きながら学ぶ看護英語の決定版。国際化時代の医療現場では英語は不可欠の時代、聞きとれること話せることは必須要素。「どうかしましたか」「どのように痛みますか」こんな会話が話せるようになる1冊。
ISBN 978-4-06-153672-2

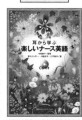

医療従事者のための 医学英語入門
清水 雅子・著
A5・216頁・定価2,750円（税込）
人体組織・器官を中心に基礎医学をコンパクトに収載した1991年刊の好評テキスト『医療技術者のための医学英語入門』が新版となって登場。図版も追加され、さらに使いやすくなった。
ISBN 978-4-06-155615-7

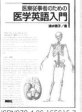

英語で学ぶプライマリーケア
西牟田 祐美子・編著
B5・112頁・定価2,200円（税込）
読んで楽しい看護学生向けテキスト。カラー4コマ漫画を手始めに、看護現場の様子を英語で学ぶことができる。リーディング、文法、演習問題も掲載。リスニング教材をホームページからダウンロード可能。
ISBN 978-4-06-520090-2

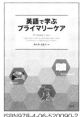

講談社サイエンティフィク　https://www.kspub.co.jp/

※表示価格は消費税（10%）が加算されています。

2021年11月現在